The Socio-Emotional Relationship Workbook for Couples

W0246418

This supportive and empowering guide helps readers identify and build on their relational values, which the dominant culture tends to minimize, inhibit, or disparage.

Written in an engaging, easy to read and use format, this workbook offers clear case examples and activities that readers can apply to their own relationships. The introductory chapter describes the problem—how unrecognized power imbalances in who notices, accommodates, and attends to one another make attaining satisfying, mutually supportive intimate relationships difficult. Chapters 2–5 introduce practices that help readers recognize the connections between their social worlds and how they engage in their relationships, with exercises that facilitate this personal awareness and enable them to share these experiences with their partners. Chapters 6–10 guide readers through assessing reciprocity in their relationships and exercises to apply each of the four components of the Circle of Care (mutual vulnerability, attunement, influence, and relational responsibility) and strategies for maintaining commitment to their relational goals over the long term. In each chapter, exercises are structured to first teach personal socio-emotional awareness, followed by relational practices that facilitate engagement based on mutual attunement and shared commitment rather than debate.

This book views emotion and meaning as the link between individuals and the larger society and helps readers develop awareness of their social contexts and societal power processes that work against relationships.

Dr. Carmen Knudson-Martin served as a director of masters and doctoral marriage, couple, and family therapy programs for 33 years and is currently professor emerita of marriage, couple, and family therapy at Lewis & Clark College in Portland, Oregon, USA.

"Partners who use this extraordinary workbook embark on a remarkable journey of depth and clarity as they develop interactions that promote a relational framework for their lives together. Carmen Knudson-Martin distills her lifetime of work as a therapist, researcher, teacher, and supervisor into practical exercises that help couples recognize cultural messages that laud the myth of individualism over egalitarian relationship-building skills—often sources of disconnection. This work emerges from watching hundreds of hours of therapy sessions both live and through scholarly coding video replays that reveal how unequal patterns in our surrounding culture affect couples' intimacy."

Douglas Huenergardt, Ph.D. Clinical Professor Loma Linda University School of Behavioral Health and Co-founder of Socio-Emotional Relationship Therapy.

"Unearned social power significantly influences our ability to cultivate security and love in intimate relationships. Sadly, books written to help couples improve their relationships rarely give this issue the attention it deserves. This highly readable and engaging workbook centralizes understanding and working through power dynamics to help couples nurture greater intimacy and connection. Dr. Knudson-Martin's warmth, wisdom, and nonjudgmental tone guide readers to meaningful self-reflection and dialogue as they begin to dismantle destructive dynamics of power in their relationship."

Tim Baima, Ph.D., LMFT.

"Recognized worldwide as a prominent figure in couple therapy, Carmen Knudson-Martin has written an insightful, timely, and practical workbook on couple relationships. Psychology and the field of couple therapy increasingly recognize that society profoundly shapes intimate relationships, often outside awareness. This relevant, engaging, and highly readable guide uniquely informs couples about what it means to care for each other and how societal forces and messages may infiltrate intimate relationships and impact emotion, intimacy, and communication, getting in the way of partners attaining the relationship they desire. This useful workbook is a must for anyone interested in understanding and strengthening their intimate relationships."

Olga Smoliak, PhD, Associate Professor, University of Guelph, Canada and a practicing psychologist and couple and family therapist.

"Carmen Knudson-Martin's workbook is a remarkable achievement, a beautiful step by step description of socio-emotional relationship therapy. It includes explanations, examples, and exercises that make visible cultural messages and assumptions about identity and hierarchy. It offers practices that help couples challenge these messages in favor of intimacy, and fosters emotional openness, responsiveness, equality and mutuality. This guide will be helpful to couple therapists as well as couples themselves."

Carol Becker, PhD, Clinical Psychologist, Therapy Training Boston, Masters Series in Couple Therapy; Public Conversations Project, and Department of Psychiatry, Harvard Medical School.

"A groundbreaking resource for couples seeking to cultivate a relationship that aligns with their values, *The Socio-Emotional Relationship Workbook for Couples* provides practical tools and insights to help overcome communication challenges and build deeper connections. This book is a must-read for anyone looking to bridge the gap between the relationship they want and the one they have."

Dr. Diane Gehart, author *Mindfulness and Acceptance in Couple and Family Therapy* and Professor, Marriage and Family Therapy, California State University Northridge.

"Although most couples desire emotional connection, too often partners struggle to recognize and overcome social influences that perpetuate power imbalances, hinder vulnerability and mutual trust, and ultimately detract from deep intimacy. Knudson-Martin's *Socio-Emotional Relationship Workbook* promotes partners' understanding of these influences and specific skills for developing self-awareness, emotional attunement, relational responsibility, and long-term commitment. This unique resource empowers partners to free themselves from roles that constrain them and co-construct the intimate and caring relationship they long for. Every couple could benefit from the vital insights and skills cultivated by this workbook."

Douglas K. Snyder, Ph.D., is Professor of Psychological and Brain Sciences at Texas A&M University (College Station) and co-author of *Getting Past the Affair and co-editor of the Clinical Handbook of Couple Therapy and What Happens in Couple Therapy: A Casebook on Effective Practice.*

The Socio-Emotional Relationship Workbook for Couples

Closing the Gap Between the Relationship You Want and the Relationship You Have

Carmen Knudson-Martin

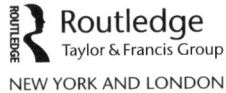
Routledge
Taylor & Francis Group

NEW YORK AND LONDON

Designed cover image: Marje © Getty Images

First published 2025
by Routledge
605 Third Avenue, New York, NY 10158

and by Routledge
4 Park Square, Milton Park, Abingdon, Oxon OX14 4RN

Routledge is an imprint of the Taylor & Francis Group, an informa business

© 2025 Carmen Knudson-Martin

The right of Carmen Knudson-Martin to be identified as author of this work has been asserted in accordance with sections 77 and 78 of the Copyright, Designs and Patents Act 1988.

All rights reserved. No part of this book may be reprinted or reproduced or utilised in any form or by any electronic, mechanical, or other means, now known or hereafter invented, including photocopying and recording, or in any information storage or retrieval system, without permission in writing from the publishers.

Trademark notice: Product or corporate names may be trademarks or registered trademarks, and are used only for identification and explanation without intent to infringe.

Access the Support Material: www.routledge.com/9781032759890

Library of Congress Cataloging-in-Publication Data
Names: Knudson-Martin, Carmen, author.
Title: The socio-emotional relationship workbook for couples : closing the gap between the relationship you want and the relationship you have / Carmen Knudson-Martin.
Description: New York, NY : Routledge, 2025. | Includes bibliographical references. |
Identifiers: LCCN 2024028192 (print) | LCCN 2024028193 (ebook) |
Subjects: LCSH: Couples therapy. | Couples–Psychology. | Interpersonal conflict.
Classification: LCC RC488.5 .K579 2025 (print) | LCC RC488.5 (ebook) |
DDC 616.89/1562–dc23/eng/20240924
LC record available at https://lccn.loc.gov/2024028192
LC ebook record available at https://lccn.loc.gov/2024028193

ISBN: 978-1-032-75993-7 (hbk)
ISBN: 978-1-032-75989-0 (pbk)
ISBN: 978-1-003-47652-8 (ebk)

DOI: 10.4324/9781003476528

Typeset in Sabon
by Taylor & Francis Books

I dedicate this book to John Knudson-Martin, my lovingly supportive life partner

Contents

Figures

Support Material

This book contains supplementary material, which can be photocopied from the back of the book. This material is also available for free digital download online. Please visit www.routledge.com/ 9781032759890 and click on the link that says "Support Material." A link to the supplementary material will appear.

Summary

Most self-help books and therapy models inadvertently locate the source of relationship problems solely within the couple or individual partners. *The Socio-Emotional Relationship Workbook for Couples* takes a different approach. It views emotion and meaning as links between individuals and the larger society and helps readers develop awareness of their social contexts and societal power processes that work against relationships. Written in an engaging, easy to read and use format, this workbook offers clear case examples and activities that readers can apply to unmask the impact of societal power processes in their lives and create the loving, two-way relationships they seek. Readers will learn:

- Socio-emotional awareness to understand yourself and your partner
- Communication skills based on mutual value and respect
- Attunement skills for emotionally connecting with your partner
- Vulnerability skills for deepening intimacy
- Practices for mutual influence and conflict resolution
- Skills for creating relationships that meet each person's needs
- Practices for sharing responsibility for the relationship
- Strategies for building trust and commitment to relational goals over the long term

Foreword by J. Maria Bermudez

This workbook is a gem! A truly unique must-have for every couple wanting a deeper and more meaningful, loving, equitable, and joyful relationship. Dr. Carmen Knudson-Martin brings to this project her life-long career as a professor, scholar, therapist, clinical supervisor, and expert in couple and family therapy. This workbook is the perfect complement to her book, *A Step-by-Step Guide to Socio-Emotional Relationship Therapy: A Socially Responsible Approach to Clinical Practice* (2024). In the event you only want to do this practice workbook, it can stand on its own, offering countless prompts to help readers have meaningful discussions. Loaded with diverse examples, it is a practical and thought-provoking guide to help you deepen your intimate connections while understanding the sociocultural forces that often block our abilities to stay attuned, supportive, and connected to one another.

This book can be used in a variety of ways. It can be read by an individual, a couple reading it together, in a clinical practicum with graduate students in training, or as a chapter-by-chapter guide for therapists conducting couple workshops or couple and marital enrichment. It will be useful to individuals and couples of any felt identity, age, or stage of relationship. The examples offer a clear description of a couple's context and the issues they are struggling with, and each vignette guides the reader to consider how to answer the questions according to their own lived experience.

At a process level, each chapter provides prompts for structured conversations for yourself or with your partner. If your partner does not participate with you, or you choose to do this workbook for your own self-awareness and growth, then you will feel guided in this process in a way that helps you make sense of your emotional responses. By answering the questions in the workbook, you will gain a deeper understanding of yourselves and greater awareness of how larger societal values, beliefs, norms, and traditions may impact how you relate to one another.

The concept of mutual attunement and the Circle of Care will be especially impactful. Carmen and I, along with Dr. Teresa McDowell, have co-authored articles and books on sociocultural attunement in family therapy, and although I am very familiar with Carmen's work, with each chapter, I found myself gaining a deeper awareness of myself and my own emotional maps. These emotional maps not only relate to my husband, children, and family but helped me think about my reactions to friends, colleagues, and my "place" at work and community, as well as the advantages and tensions I hold related to different aspects of my identity. Reading the examples of different couples was helpful and thought-provoking to me.

This workbook is truly a pleasure to read, especially if you read it with an open mind and heart and a willingness to gain a deeper awareness of yourself in relation to others. You will also learn more about how we are all impacted by societal pressures that affect our sense of self and how we navigate our relationships. As Dr. Knudson-Martin states in Chapter 4, "This awareness will help you recognize and appreciate what is important to you, see how *what* you feel connects to your relationships and place in the world, and use this awareness to improve your relational connections."

While written in an accessible and clear manner, each chapter is grounded in sound research on how social norms, values and rules, power dynamics, biological processes, and different types of vulnerabilities affect our minds and relationships. Reading each vignette and peeking into the dynamics of diverse couples allows the opportunity to compare your reactions to the experiences of the couples used as examples.

At the end of each chapter, readers are guided to orient to each other and calmly answer reflexive questions that help deepen self and other awareness related to the chapter topic, creating rich dialog opportunities that will undoubtedly be beneficial. Readers are also given additional resources to better understand the chapter's key topic and suggestions for integrating the corresponding handout/activity at the end of the book in the appendices.

I will certainly recommend this workbook to all the couples I know and to every couple I work with in therapy. Many of my clients seek couple therapy for problems related to communication, emotional distance, and resentment. Once they can turn toward each other and communicate with attunement and commitment, they can safely say what is on their minds and hearts in ways that strengthen their relationship. I am confident that if a couple reads this book together and practices the components of it daily, they will enrich their relationship. While the perfect companion for couples therapy, this workbook will help couples engage in a deeply meaningful experience even if they are not in counseling. With commitment and focus, the rewards can be great and enduring.

As Dr. Knudson-Martin so eloquently states in Chapter 6, "Doing the activities and conversations in this book means you have already been taking steps toward mutual vulnerability. You have shown openness to learning about your sensitivities and curiosity about your partner's experience. You are willing to try something new."

Whatever you do… do not abandon the workbook after the first few chapters. It is outstanding, and you will want to complete the book and do the activities until the very end… no matter how long it takes for you to do it. It is well worth it! I also recommend that you go over it at least once a year, like a relational wellness check. If an ounce of prevention is worth a pound of cure, then completing this workbook is certainly more enjoyable and worth investing in than the time and money it will take for you to engage in crisis intervention after years of not nurturing the wellness of your relationship. As Dr. Knudson-Martin writes, "mutual attunement and shared relational responsibility is a two-way street and very important for a healthy and loving relationship."

J. Maria Bermudez, PhD., LMFT, is an Associate Professor of Human Development and Family Science and Couple and Family Therapy at the University of Georgia. She is a Clinical Fellow and an Approved Supervisor of the American Association of Family Therapy and co-author of *Socioculturally Attuned Family Therapy: Guidelines for Equitable Theory and Practice* (2018, 2023).

Background and Acknowledgments

This workbook translates the components of Socio-Emotional Relationship Therapy (SERT) into practical steps that can be used by anyone. Identifying the gap between the relationship couples want and the relationships most have was the result of research with Anne Rankin Mahoney. Together with a team of doctoral students, we set out to learn what was happening inside couple relationships across the globe and lifespan. Anne's dedication to research that shows not only what is happening, but why, her insistence on clear writing, and her collaborative approach are reflected in everything I have done since.

Developing SERT was catalyzed by the happy accident of working with Douglas Huenergardt at Loma Linda University. As a result of our shared interest in gender, culture, and power in couple therapy, we formed a clinical research team to study our own practices and determine what works. Over fifteen years, more than 60 different clinician-researchers helped articulate Socio-Emotional Relationship Therapy and publish the research upon which it is founded. Lana Kim, my colleague at the Lewis & Clark, has been impactful in seeing SERT as an intervention into social narratives that prioritize individuality at the expense of relationships. Lana also pushes me to continually expand our understanding of culture and the "felt" nature of our social identities.

My awareness of the influence of sociocultural and larger systems further evolved as I worked with Teresa McDowell and Maria Bermudez to develop *Socioculturally Attuned Family Therapy: Guidelines for Equitable Theory and Practice,* now in its second edition. Our generative conversations have contributed immeasurably to the practices presented here. This book also draws on much of the best thinking in marital, couple, and family therapy. Citations to many of these works may be found in *A Step-by-Step Guide to Socio-Emotional Relationship Therapy: A Socially Responsible Approach to Clinical Practice.* The format for conversations used throughout the book is adapted from the practices for addressing divisive topics in a non-polarizing, relational way developed by the Public Conversations Project in Boston.

Most of all, I am grateful to the countless couples who have opened their hearts and lives to my colleagues and me in therapy and research. The examples in this book come from their life stories. Their names and circumstances are changed to protect their identities, but their hopes and struggles are very real. And, like you, I live in a particular sociocultural context with people I love and care about. My husband John, son Chris, daughter Kyara, their partners Melanie and Jerome, and grandsons Ethan and Kai are most dear to me. I am grateful for their love and the joy and promise their lives bring.

I developed this book with you in mind—that you will feel less alone or confused about the struggles you face, and that the ideas and practices in each chapter will help you evolve the loving, mutually supportive relationships you want.

Author Bio

Carmen Knudson-Martin, PhD, LMFT, is Professor Emerita of the Marital, Couple, and Family Therapy Program at Lewis & Clark College, Portland OR, USA and a founder of Socio-Emotional Relationship Therapy. Carmen has published over 100 articles and book chapters on the influence of the larger sociocultural context in couple and family relationships and the political and ethical implications of therapist actions on marital equality, relational development, and couple therapy. She is editor/author of five other books, including *A Step-by-Step guide to Socio-Emotional Relationship Therapy: A Socially Responsible Approach to Clinical Practice* (Routledge, 2024) and *Socioculturally Attuned Family Therapy: Guidelines for Equitable Theory and Practice, 2nd Ed.* (Routledge, 2023). Carmen was the 2017 recipient of the Distinguished Contribution to Family Therapy Theory and Practice award from the American Family Therapy Academy.

Chapter 1

Why so Many Relationships Fail—and the Secret to Success

When my colleagues and I asked couples what a good relationship looks like, nearly all described the same expectation—whether in their first years together, raising teenagers or retired, they imagined open communication and being there for each other. Yet as we explored what actually happens in their relationships, most fell short of these ideals. Without realizing they were doing so, they fell into patterns that limit connection and create an imbalance in whose needs and interests are centered.

Example

Mark and Lisa are in their first year of marriage. Lisa was attracted to Mark because he "shows his feminine side" and respected her career. Mark liked that Lisa is assertive and he expects both of them to be involved in home life, to have careers, and to grow personally. But when asked how they decide how to spend time together, Lisa says, "if I know Mark is going to be home, then I prioritize being together and do not plan something else that night." In contrast, Mark responds, "It would really upset me if she made plans for us and told me 'We're doing this'."

Lisa orients to Mark and their relationship, while Mark emphasizes independence and control over his activities. Over time, their life together becomes structured around Mark's schedule and interests, which is reflected in their communication:

Mark and Lisa approach communication from different positions—she is more focused on him and his well-being than he is on her. Mark: "I expect to be listened to and supported... [and] it is not my role to make Lisa happy." Lisa: "I can be overly sensitive. I try to be supportive of Mark and less reactive to my emotions."

Why Power Imbalances are a Relationship Problem

Though Mark and Lisa believe in a two-way flow between them, the difference in who is oriented to whom is part of larger societal patterns that emphasize individuality and create unintended power imbalances in whose interests are treated as important and who is attending to the relationship. This gap between the loving, mutually supportive relationships couples say they want and what they *do* shows up time and again. The imbalance creates trouble communicating, limits emotional connection, and makes it difficult to address conflict or creatively adapt to stress and life changes. It also contributes to mental health problems such as anxiety and depression.

Power differences are like toxins in the air; they are harmful but can be hard to see. They influence how you feel, show your love, and communicate. They interact with the ways you were raised and how you come to know yourself and others. While especially difficult for heterosexual/different gender couples to recognize, power inequities happen in all kinds of relationships. They occur even though you want your relationships to mutually support and benefit each of you.

DOI: 10.4324/9781003476528-1

Below are indicators of a likely power imbalance. Which might apply to you?

- ❑ Awareness of the other is not equal
- ❑ It is not safe to be vulnerable, creating emotional distance
- ❑ Communication and openness to influence are limited
- ❑ The needs and interests of the less powerful partner are overlooked
- ❑ Conflict is almost impossible to address
- ❑ Responsibility for maintaining the relationship is not shared
- ❑ Options during times of stress or change are restricted
- ❑ You feel hopeless that problems can be resolved
- ❑ Intimacy and emotional connection are thwarted
- ❑ Love withers

Creating a Path to Mutuality

Why are loving, mutually supportive relationships so elusive? Why do so many good people struggle to create the kind of relationships they want? To answer this question and find solutions, our research group studied the exceptions—couples who are able to make their relational dreams real. We learned that this is not just an interpersonal problem; it is also a societal problem. Simply put, you live in a society that works against relationships. We learned how some people overcome these barriers to stay emotionally connected and support each other—to negotiate life together rather than be pulled apart. This book will show you how.

Our journey together will be based on Socio-Emotional Relationship Therapy (SERT), an approach that helps you counteract the destructive effects of gender, culture, and power and create relationships based on mutual care and support. In this chapter you will learn to recognize the foundations of good relationships and why they can be so hard to attain. You will discover the secret to moving beyond these obstacles and how to use the chapters that follow to improve communication and create a more consciously connected, mutually satisfying and loving relationship.

What is a Good Relationship?

The people we interviewed intuitively understood that good relationships are a *two-way street* in which partners communicate and emotionally connect with each other. I think of this as the two Rs:

- ✓ Reciprocity—care and support go back and forth relatively equally
- ✓ Responsivity—partners are aware of and respond to each other's needs

Relationship science backs this up. All of us, whatever our age, *need* to both "feel felt" and to be aware of others. Interpersonal neurobiologists call this attunement. It means getting on each other's wavelength, or as my colleague Jessica ChenFeng described, it is like tuning a guitar, "if the tuning isn't right on pitch, then it's not tuned. Both the guitar and the tuning fork must be on the same note" (Pandit et al., 2014, p. 74).

This felt sense of emotional fittedness is necessary for healthy human development. As a child, you needed it to manage your emotions and develop a sense that it is safe to step into the larger world. Your need for this kind of emotional connection is lifelong. When others attune to you and you attune to them, you experience a sense of belonging and that you matter. This is an essential component of physical and emotional health.

> **Supportive relational connections are as important to your health as whether or not you smoke (U.S. Surgeon General advisory on the healing effects of social connection and community, 2023).**

No one is able to be on the same wavelength all the time. Conflict, disagreement, and even hurt are part of all relationships. But mutually supportive partners approach these with responsibility for the well-being of their partners in mind, as well as their own. This means you are curious about your partner's perspective and open to being influenced. When a rupture occurs in your relationship, you are equally likely to initiate repair.

Your need for connection and community is not limited to intimate and family relationships. It extends to your sense of worth, value, and belongingness in the larger society. The developmental psychologist Allan Schore (2021) stated it well:

> *Throughout life interpersonal synchrony, operating beneath levels of awareness, acts as a fundamental interpersonal neurobiological mechanism not only within dyads, but also in all human group dynamics, and in the organization of all cultures.*
>
> (p. 12)

Your experience of support, belonging, and worth in the larger society affects, and is affected by, your ability to form and maintain loving, mutually supportive close relationships.

Example

> *Judith and Janelle have been together for three years and are thinking about getting married. They were attracted because they understood each other's struggles with mental health and had fun together. But Judith is worried she cannot trust Janelle because she spends so much time with friends and recently lent a friend money without telling her. As the couple developed awareness of their experiences in the larger society, their struggle with trust made more sense. Both grew up in low-income families and communities that did not understand or attune to their experiences of sexuality and gender. Their parents faced discrimination and financial stresses that added to their struggles. Judith responded by learning to depend on herself and not need others. Janelle learned to smile and keep things smooth by focusing on what others need. When they met, Judith was "blown away" by how interested Janelle was in her. Janelle was "fascinated" by Judith, who seemed confident and knew what she wanted.*

Janelle and Judith began their relationship with an imbalance in who attended to and focused on the other—an imbalance resulting from their different responses to a world where people were not open to their queer experiences and neither could feel felt.

Neither had learned what to expect in a two-way, mutually supportive relationship. Once they do, each can take responsibility for improving the flow of power between them and building trust.

How do the Characteristics of a Mutually Supportive Relationship Apply to You?

❑ My partner and I are usually on each other's wavelength
❑ I feel felt in my relationship
❑ My partner and I reciprocally respond to each other
❑ I experience emotional connection and intimacy with my partner
❑ My relationship supports my sense of worth, safety, and belonging
❑ My health is enhanced by the two-way nature of my relationship
❑ My emotional connection with my partner helps me respond to challenges and stress in the larger world
❑ My partner is attentive to my well-being
❑ Each of us seeks to repair ruptures in our relationship

Which of the above statements are especially meaningful to you? Why?

_____

_____

_____

_____

_____

_____

_____

_____

How the Social World Works Against Relationships

When your relationship is not working, it is easy to blame yourself or your partner—or both. You may think something is wrong with you. You may wonder what you have a right to expect and what you should give. Despite intuitively knowing this balance should be fair and life-enhancing, most people do not have a model of what a mutually supportive relationship actually looks like. As a society, our ideals about marriage and other intimate relationships have changed faster than our behaviors. Knowing how society affects you and your partner helps close this gap.

With the help of the Figure 1.1, picture yourself within a web of relationships extending from your closest intimate relationships to other family and friends. These are embedded within your community (workplace, school, church, other associations), and all these are connected to the larger society (cultural, social, political, and economic systems). This is the relational you, with connections going back and forth between each level. If you are like most people, you experience yourself, your close relationships, and work and family roles personally without much awareness of the impact of the bigger social picture.

Social forces influence your day-to-day life in three ways. The examples of Mark and Lisa and Judith and Janelle illustrate how.

1 Society defines who and what is important

As North Americans, both couples live in a world that prioritizes individualism and monetary success. Characteristics such as assertiveness, competitiveness, independence, and decisiveness are valued more than empathy, cooperativeness, openness to multiple perspectives, or caring for others. Each partner has learned these societal messages about what is important. As the ones more focused on their partners, Lisa and Janelle receive strong messages that they *should* be more independent, clearer about what they want. At the same time, though in different settings, each learned that the quality of their relationships is their responsibility. When there is "miscommunication," they tend to automatically blame themselves and try to be more careful about how they communicate.

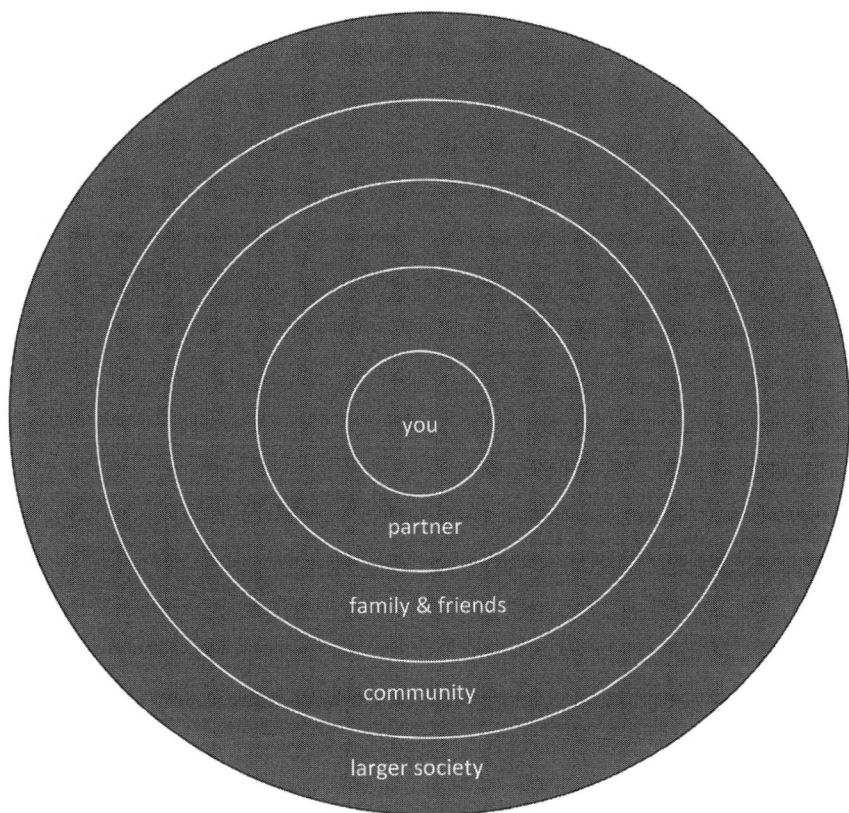

you

partner

family & friends

community

larger society

Figure 1.1 The relational you.

For their part, Mark and Judith demonstrate socially valued characteristics of independence and self-reliance and are less likely to focus on the relationship or assume responsibility for relational problems. They see their partners as overly reactive or needing to learn to better express themselves. Yet, when you ask them, both Mark and Judith care about their partners and want what is best for them.

In any society, those in more powerful positions determine which characteristics and values are important. Over time, these become built into social norms: how families and workplaces operate, whose voice is viewed credible, and whose worth is validated. When Lisa automatically organizes her life according to Mark's schedule, she repeats societal messages that men's time is more valuable than women's. Judith and Janelle receive social messages that their sexualities are "different" or "deviant" from the mainstream. As "poor" children from families with fewer economic resources, each also received messages that they are less worthy than their more affluent classmates.

Whether or not you agree with dominant societal values, they affect everyone. We all live in a world where some voices and ways of being are valued more than others.

When you hear "success," what are the first words that pop into your mind?

Do your ideas about success fit dominant societal values or resist them? How?

_____

_____

_____

_____

2 Emotion reflects your experience in the world

Emotions are important. They are your body's read of the social environment and a means for communicating with yourself and others. What stimulates your emotion depends on the social/interpersonal meaning in the situation. For example, when Mark is upset at a plan Lisa made, Lisa gets a lump in her throat, has a hard time breathing, and feels guilty. Her emotional response reflects the gendered rule that she should keep Mark happy; if he is not, it is her fault. When Judith sees Janelle spend "too much" time with friends, her chest gets tight, she breathes faster, and feels angry. Her reaction arises within persistent societal messages that denigrate her and tell her she is not important.

3 Societal power imbalances limit intimate relationships

Your gender, sexuality, race, socio-economic status, and many other positions in society carry varying degrees of social power that contribute to your ability to influence your world. Power imbalances in the larger society influence other developmental processes and affect how you judge yourself and your partner and how you emotionally connect, communicate, and resolve conflict. When power is not equal intimacy is thwarted. If you are in a powerful position, you cannot let weakness or uncertainty show; if you have less power, you have to guard what you say to protect yourself, calm your partner, and maintain your relationships.

In line with what he learned as a White male, Mark feels free to express anger when upset. Lisa (who learned women are responsible for maintaining relationships) usually responds by trying to soothe him and/or changing her behavior. Sometimes Lisa also expresses upset or anger. When she does, Mark (whose male socialization pressures him to get things "right") feels criticized and responds with anger. Lisa feels guilty for creating the disruption and inadequate for not "communicating better." These are "natural" interpersonal responses to enacting societally gendered power imbalances. It is not what either Mark or Lisa wants. If this pattern continues, unproductive fights will escalate, or one or both will emotionally (and even physically) distance to avoid conflict or hurt.

Even as much has changed, gendered power imbalances are surprisingly persistent, both in intimate relationships and in the larger society. Now, they are often more subtle and harder to see. For example, Lisa and Mark are both nurses. They share most housework, enjoy each other's company, and often have "good" conversations on a variety of topics. They are puzzled and distressed by the growing gap between them.

Gender is only one of many societal power processes that infect intimate relationships. Societal messages that tell Judith and Janelle they are "less than" increase the vulnerability they bring to their relationship. While shared experiences of distress and discrimination draw them together, their vulnerability in the larger world increases the pressure on their relationship and makes trust more difficult. To Judith, Janelle is all she has in a hostile world. Her vulnerable position makes her want to rein Janelle in, keep her close. To Janelle, other relationships are a life line for which she is responsible. Though Judith and Janelle talk about many aspects of their lives, their differing responses to family stress and social marginalization stimulate intense emotions and make each feel unsafe. They want to pull together, trust, and support each other, but are sometimes at a loss for how to do so.

What obstacles to connection and mutual support come up in your relationship?

_____

_____

_____

_____

_____

In my work with couples, I am fascinated by how so many aspects of each person's background and life experience come together. When problems arise, it can be like Velcro—each side seems to reach out and grab the other to keep you stuck, trapped in painful patterns you don't want. Many factors are involved. Some challenges are more complex than others. But whatever struggles and stressors you face, your way through them is easier with a foundation of mutual care and support.

How to Overcome Obstacles to Mutually Supportive Relationships

In our research, three behaviors distinguish couples who attain mutually supportive relationships:

- Conscious "we" focus
- Intentional action
- Openness to learning

While other couples do what feels natural and fall into inequitable relationship patterns without discussion, mutually supportive couples consciously prioritize their relational values. You are aware of obstacles such as societal expectations that women are better at dealing with emotions or that being influenced by others is a sign of weakness, and discuss how you want your relationships to work. Rather than automatically doing what each is good at, you are willing to learn new ways of relating. Even though it is sometimes uncomfortable, you make room for each voice and learn from and address the conflict that may result.

Example

Jen and Rob have a clear vision of what mutuality means to them. Their written promise hangs on their wall: "We will share equally the rewards of the relationship and respect each other's need for mutual nurturing." Each partner is attentive to the flow of power. Rob: "It isn't something that is just done by rote … Jen will say I don't like this, or this is getting unbalanced. Or I will say this is getting unbalanced.
(Knudson-Martin & Mahoney, 2009, pp. 48–56)

Emotional connection and mutual support seldom "just happen." You need socio-emotional awareness, conscious intention, and openness.

When Jen suggests a change to a backyard project Rob is working on, he first feels a stab of criticism, like he's done something wrong. But he recognizes this as a response to societal gender *messages that tell him that he should be in charge and know what he's doing. Instead of a "natural" gruff reaction that would hurt Jen, he looks at her and says, "tell me more about what you're thinking." He prioritizes their "we."*

Reading this book suggests you want to make an intentional commitment to "we." With your willingness to learn, the exercises in this book will help you:

❑   Develop a clear vision of your relational goals
❑   Build socio-emotional awareness that helps you recognize how societal forces affect what you feel and do
❑   Take intentional action to overcome barriers to connection and mutual support
❑   Practice the Circle of Care, including mutual vulnerability, attunement, influence, and relational responsibility
❑   Draw on your relational values in times of stress and change

How to Use this Book

The exercises in this book invite you to slow down, to breathe, and to learn about yourself, your partner, your relationship, and the world around you. The goals are awareness and learning how to support each other.

Each chapter includes exercises that involve personal self-reflection followed by a conversational activity. Your learning will be better if you share the journey with someone. If your partner is willing to participate with you, this is ideal. If your intimate relationship is not at a place where this is possible or if it feels unsafe, doing the exercises with a friend or in a group will also be valuable. It is also possible to benefit from the exercises individually. This will give you the chance to reflect on yourself and what you want in a relationship. It can be an opportunity to practice being how you want to be in a relationship and to see what happens. If doing the exercises on your own (or with your partner) is difficult or stressful, doing them with the aid of a therapist or counselor that focuses on the systemic nature of relationships will be helpful.

Let's get started.

Orienting Exercise

Practice this exercise several times, until you are familiar with it. Repeat it before beginning the exercises in each of the chapters that follow.

1   Make yourself comfortable and close your eyes.
2   Be aware of your breath as it gently goes in and out.
3   Picture yourself in the center of a small circle. Be aware of any tension, worry, or judgment. Gently let them go.

   a   Expand your circle to include your partner(s). Be aware of any tension, worry, or judgment. Gently let them go.
   b   Expand your circle to include family and friends. Be aware of any tension, worry, or judgment. Gently let them go.
   c   Expand your circle to include your community, your workplace or school, your church or other meaningful associations. Be aware of any tension, worry, or judgment. Gently let them go.
   d   Expand your circle to include the larger society. Be aware of any tension, worry, or judgment. Gently let them go.

4   Be aware of your breath going in and out.
5   Commit to compassion for yourself and your partner and curiosity to learn.

What is it like to expand your circle of self?

_____

_____

_____

What is it like to take a curious, non-judgmental position?

_____

_____

_____

Conversation 1

This exercise introduces the format for the conversational activities in this book. They begin with a personal story or experience, invite you to reflect on questions and uncertainties, and end with new thoughts and commitments. The key is to listen and learn, rather than debate.

Instructions:

- One person responds to the first question for up to two minutes. The listener does not comment. Then the other person (or persons) also takes up to two minutes to respond to the first question, while the other(s) listens without comment.
- Repeat for each question, alternating who begins.
- If you are doing the exercise without a partner, write your answers and then read them aloud to yourself. (_Hearing your own voice is important._)
- There are no "right" answers.
- When speaking, give yourself time to let your thoughts unfold.
- When listening, focus on the other person's experience. When your focus slips to your reaction, gently return your focus to the speaker. (_It is very important to not interrupt or comment._)

1   Share a story about good couple relationships that is meaningful to you.

2   Share a story that motivates you to engage in the exercises in this workbook.

3   When it comes to relationships that mutually support each partner, what are you uncertain or confused about?

4   As you listen to your partner, what would you like to better understand or know more about? (_Partner does not answer these questions._)

5   As you engage in this conversation, what new ideas or questions come up for you?

6   What personal commitment will you carry forward as you complete this relationship journey?

Additional Resources

The relational you. Make copies of this diagram from Appendix A at the back of this book or download online by visiting www.routledge.com/9781032759890 and clicking on the link that says "Support Material." Personalize your diagram by writing in the names of the people, groups, and kinds of communities and larger social forces that make up your relational world. You can also complete one from your childhood and compare with your partner. Discussing these diagrams with your partner or others will increase your relational awareness and help your journey toward the relationship you want.

More on Socio-Emotional Relationship Therapy (SERT). SERT is the outgrowth of decades of research. Anne Mahoney and I, together with an international team of researchers, began by interviewing couples across cultures and life stages about their relationships. We were especially interested in how they managed the influences of gender and power. For a collection of these studies see *Couples, Gender, and Power: Creating Change in Intimate Relationships* (Knudson-Martin & Mahoney, 2009). This research identified the gap between the relationships couples want and the relationships they have, and drew attention to mutual support and the Circle of Care as critical outcomes in efforts to help couples.

Building on these studies, Douglas Huenergardt and I formed a research group to study our practice of couple therapy as we worked with issues related to gender, culture, and power. Our focus was "what works" to help people develop relational possibilities beyond the limits of dominant individualistic, patriarchal social legacies. In collaboration with co-investigator Lana Kim, over 60 clinician-researchers participated in our research teams. The findings have been published in numerous academic journals. For an integration of these studies, case illustrations, practical clinical guidelines, and references to related works, see *A Step-by-Step Guide to Socio-Emotional Relationship Therapy: A Socially Responsible Approach to Clinical Practice* (Knudson-Martin, 2024).

Chapter 2

Center Relationships

What matters to you? Making money? Success in your job? Being healthy? Paying the bills? You probably say family and close relationships top your list. But relational fitness does not come automatically, and your relational hopes and skills are not what the larger society judges important or views as markers of success. Modern culture is not organized to sustain loving relationships. Yet study after study shows that relationships are what make us thrive. In fact, Harvard researchers Robert Waldinger and Marc Schultz (2023) boil down all their years of study to one principle: "*Good relationships keep us healthier and happier. Period*" (p. 10). The happiest people center relationships.

In this chapter you will take a closer look at your relational values and goals. You will learn why it is important to consciously center them and how to recognize societal forces that work against you. To help you prioritize and practice your relational values, you'll be introduced to the Circle of Care—four orienting principles that promote mutually supportive, health-enhancing relationships.

We will use the example of Jason and Rebecca to illustrate how to center relationships. This heterosexual couple initially followed what was expected in a society oriented toward productivity and "success." Their experience highlights common relational challenges in a culture that promotes disconnection.

> *Jason and Rebecca have been together for over 30 years and married for 23. But they nearly separated after five years and hit another crisis eight years later when Rebecca was feeling overwhelmed and depressed. At that time, Rebecca sought help from a therapist who helped her and Jason identify their relational values and apply the Circle of Care. Since then, their relationship not only remains strong; their base of mutual support helps them flourish, despite facing several major life challenges.*

The Culture of Disconnection

Rebecca and Jason met at work—their first jobs since completing degrees in public administration (Rebecca) and business management (Jason). Oriented toward achievement, they worked long hours and often joined each other for something to eat after a busy day. They discovered a common passion for the outdoors and started hiking together on weekends. After a while, it "made sense" to move in together. They shared many interests and friends and respected each's personal goals, activities, and work responsibilities; however, societal messages that promote disconnection, competition, and isolation at the expense of relationship nearly broke them apart. How did that happen?

Look at the lists of qualities below? Which do you think society values most? Which do you value most?

❑	Self-directed	❑	Empathic
❑	Assertive	❑	Collaborative
❑	Independent	❑	Listener
❑	Strong	❑	Sensitive
❑	In control	❑	Flexible
❑	Rational	❑	Emotionally attuned
❑	Competitive	❑	Humble
❑	Productive	❑	Nurturing
❑	Decisive	❑	Open

DOI: 10.4324/9781003476528-2

None of these qualities in and of themselves are bad. But the qualities in the list on the left tend to be valued in modern culture, while the qualities on the right are minimized or denigrated. Jason and Rebecca are immersed in a work and social environment that emphasizes the left list and a culture of self-sufficiency and dominance that suppresses human connection in every aspect of life. It tells you that to get ahead, you need to know what you want, be assertive, and project your strength. Though in actuality traits such as humility, warmth, and empathy are associated with well-functioning workplaces and relationships, Rebecca and Jason learned early on that these were not the qualities that would be respected and rewarded.

Look at these lists again. Think of the left list as examples of a culture of disconnection and domination. The right list exemplifies qualities that build relationship, that nurture well-being, happiness, and health, and as relational experts Saliha Bava and Mark Greene (2023) put it, *"are the lifeblood for successful organizations, communities, and families alike"* (p. 12). We are born with the capacity for these relational qualities. In fact, people who study human development find that young children—boys, as well as girls—regularly demonstrate them (Way et al., 2018). But as we grow older, these relational qualities tend not to be socially reinforced. The social degradation of relationality affects everyone, but may be experienced differently depending on your gender and other social factors.

Five years into their relationship, Rebecca is offered what she considers a "dream position." But it would involve moving. She is also feeling the "biological clock." These life choices necessarily involve Jason, but when they try to discuss them, they run into an impasse:

REBECCA: I'm excited about this new job possibility. It's what I always hoped to do.

JASON: I would never stand in the way of the job of your dreams. But my life is here. It's your choice. I'll understand if you go.

REBECCA: (*hurt that Jason doesn't seem willing to talk about moving with her, but feeling responsible for the relationship*) I would never ask you to give up your job. And I'd like to have kids someday— that would be hard if we're living apart.

JASON: (*sighs and sounds a bit irritated*) I think you have to decide what you want. I'd like kids too, but it's really your choice. I'll support you either way.

Rebecca leaves the conversation feeling torn between her relational desires and her career. Since they have not been able to discuss and explore the complexities involved for each of them, she feels disconnected from Jason and turns to friends to help work through "her" choice. Jason feels disconnected as well. He is embarrassed by the anxiety he feels at the thought that Rebecca might leave. He wants to support her, but doesn't know how. The subject makes him feel incompetent and out of control, so he avoids it. When Rebecca says she decided to turn down the job, he is relieved. They decide to marry and begin thinking about having a family.

Choices like these are complicated, with no one "right" answer. The problem is not with the decisions; the problem is with *how* they were made. Jason and Rebecca's conversation was dominated by social messages that privilege individual choice and emphasize personal achievements without a way to prioritize their shared relational interests. Lacking a relational model to guide them, they fell into common patterns that value men's work over women's and placed unacknowledged responsibility for maintaining the relationship on Rebecca, while leaving them disconnected from each other.

Rebecca and Jason developed their initial relationship patterns around workplace demands and their culturally reinforced emphasis on personal goals and space. Though they cared a lot about each other, they did not have a model for how to build and prioritize their "we." As a result, when faced with conflict and change, they automatically replicated societal-based gender stereotypes.

(Un)Learning Disconnection Culture

Stereotypic gender messages are woven into the broader disconnection culture. You learn them in school as you interact with other children and through what is modeled and portrayed in media and people around you. Boys are hit especially early. If you identify as male you learn you need to be strong; being "weak" is forbidden and expressing emotion or needing others means you're weak. If you identify as female, beginning as a teenager, you learn to protect relationships by hiding or minimizing aspects of yourself. Many young women learn that to be successful they need to act "more like a man" and hide (or overcome) their relational interests. Not everyone responds to these societal messages in the same way, but they affect you and your relationships nonetheless. If you identify as non-binary or transgender, you necessarily confront them early on.

What these "old" gender messages look like in modern life can be hard to see. For example, it was important to Jason to not dominate Rebecca. His reaction to the relational bind provoked by her job offer was to "support her" by [unconsciously] prioritizing individualism, which distanced him from her and his own relational needs. And, even as she "chose" to maintain the relationship, Rebecca closed down parts of herself, keeping them outside the relationship and lost to both of them. Their communication and emotional connection were thwarted, despite their genuine joy in deciding to marry and have children.

Both Jason and Rebecca had absorbed individualistic culture ideas about success and worth (i.e., maturity and leadership mean being self-directed, assertive, independent, strong, in control, rational, competitive, productive, decisive). If asked, Rebecca and Jason also valued relational characteristics (such as empathy, collaboration, listening, sensitivity, flexibility, emotional attunement, humility, nurturance, openness), but few cultural messages support these relational ideas, equating them instead with femininity, weakness, and lack of direction. Both partners experienced internal conflict regarding these competing value systems, but they did not have words or awareness through which to helpfully address them.

Think about the messages regarding relational qualities (empathy, flexibility, emotional attunement, humility, etc.) in your world. List as many as you can in the space below. Write whatever comes up for you. Do not worry about whether they are "right."

_____

_____

_____

_____

_____

What do these messages say about what you *should* do? What is good or expected?

_____

_____

_____

You live in a world with many different messages. Some carry more weight or social value than others. They represent different value systems and priorities, with differing impacts on what is possible and ideal in your relationships. Most likely, you receive mixed or competing messages, but like Jason and Rebecca, seldom have the opportunity to reflect on them.

Think about the sources of the messages you listed. Where did they come from? If they came from your family or friends, where do you think they got them?

_____

_____

_____

How do these messages affect how you judge yourself and relate to your partner and others close to you?

_____

_____

_____

Who or what do these messages benefit? How well do they work for you?

_____

_____

_____

Which relational values do you want to prioritize?

_____

_____

_____

What relational values are missing that you would like to add or expand upon?

_____

_____

_____

The more you look for your relational values and recognize the societal messages that work against or support them, the more relational possibilities you will have. Knowing how your relationships, health, and well-being work together will help you envision and clarify your relational goals.

Born to Connect

You were born into a web of connections. As human, you necessarily have to read, respond, and adapt to the world around you. Your ability to attune to and take in the experience of others is critical. And others need to know and understand you. Well-being depends on mutual openness and responsiveness. Even as infants, this connection is a two-way street. Consider this example with Jason and their infant daughter, Alesia:

> *As Jason begins to put Alesia to bed, she reaches up and grabs his hair. Jason responds with a grimace and loud "Ouch!!" Alesia looks away and screws up her face. Jason senses her distress and immediately responds, soothing her hair and talking softly to calm her. After a few moments, Alesia looks at him and smiles. Jason returns her smile.*

In this two-way dance of relational rupture and reconnection, Alesia is able to have an impact on her father and he responds with care. This is how you learn to trust. The openness and responsiveness Jason demonstrates is a necessary lifelong orientation to others that builds and maintains supportive relationships. On a neurobiological level, your neurons literally take in and mirror another's experience, to be "with." This relational circuit not only enables each of you to feel felt; it catalyzes hope, possibility, and creative response to life's challenges.

Many factors can interact with societal messages to limit your openness and receptivity to others. As children, Jason and Rebecca each experienced love and safety in their families. If you experienced trauma such as child abuse, bullying, or sexual/physical assault or live with ongoing, day-to-day discrimination or marginalization that tells you that you and people like you are not welcome or valued, or you have experienced the sociocultural trauma of war or political oppression, it is harder to be open. To escape pain, your body may shut down mechanisms for human connection. When this happens, and/or you have been socialized to not need others, you are deprived of the relational lifeblood you need to thrive. As Judith Herman (2023), the noted expert on trauma and recovery, stated, "[you] cannot feel safe alone" (p. 2). The impact of the challenges and traumas you face depends on relationships that take in and are moved by your experience, who join with you to create shared meaning that honors and validates you.

When openness and responsiveness are not mutual, connection is thwarted and even daily routines and activities can take their toll. This is what happened to Rebecca and Jason.

> *In their eighth year of marriage, Rebecca is the director of a local foodbank. She loves her work and the people they serve. Jason is well-established in his career as sales manager for a local company. Both are loving and responsive parents of a two-year-old and five-year-old. But Rebecca is feeling overwhelmed, stressed, and depressed. She wonders what is wrong with her? Why can't she cope better and appreciate the many blessings in her life? When she calls a therapist to help manage her stress, the therapist invites Jason to the first session. In the brief segments of their conversation below, the therapist explores the nature of their bond, with an eye toward reciprocity:*

THERAPIST: How would you describe your connection with each other?

JASON: It's good. I think we communicate better than most couples.

REBECCA: (*softly*) We're good. I especially appreciate that Jason is good with the kids. He's a good dad.

THERAPIST: (*highlights a difference in well-being*) Jason, I notice that you appear to be doing well, have lots of energy, while Rebecca seems worn out, worrying that she cannot cope. How do you think this difference happens?

JASON: Rebecca works too hard. People are always asking things of her. She needs better boundaries—needs to take better care of herself.

REBECCA: (*sits up straighter, speaks with energy*) When I have a day off, I spend it with the kids and taking care of the house. When you have a day off, you go fishing or golfing!

This opens a conversation about relational goals, fairness, and their responsibilities to each other and their family that Jason and Rebecca never had before. Over the years they had fallen into patterns that avoided conflict but limited reciprocity and mutual well-being. When they discussed what was happening, they were able to make changes based on their egalitarian relationship values and fairness. Rebecca's stress and symptoms of depression abated.

When Rebecca and Jason saw the imbalance in their relationship, they were both clear that they did not want their relationship to support Jason at Rebecca's expense and that this also kept them more disconnected from each other than they wanted. Their first step was to identify their relational needs and values. Take a moment to reflect on these in your life.

Given that humans are born to need each other, what are some of your relational needs?

What is it like for you when your partner (or others) seems to "get" what you are experiencing?

What is it like for you when you are able to connect with what your partner (or others) is experiencing?

What is it like when you feel disconnected? That your partner (or others) doesn't have a sense of what it is like to be you?

When you think about how you want your relationship to work, what is important to you?

_____

_____

_____

The Invisibility of Caring

For generations, the effort that goes into caring for and about others has been overlooked—hidden and made invisible, not valued or noticed. Centering relationships means that you acknowledge and value care work, such as:

- Effort spent noticing how others are doing and offering aid and support
- Thinking about what is needed for your relationships and the well-being of those you love
- Keeping track of schedules and planning for what your family and partner need
- Doing the behind the scenes work that keeps a home running smoothly
- The mental "to-do" list of all that your family and partner need

Rebecca had been doing most of this care work. Since it was not noticed, valued, and shared, she felt exhausted and incompetent. Jason thought of himself as a family man, but had not learned to recognize and center the value of care. Valuing care work is part of an approach to relationships we call the Circle of Care.

The Circle of Care

Like most couples today, Jason and Rebecca wanted a mutually supportive relationship, but did not have a vision of what that would look like. The therapist introduced them to the Circle of Care—four orienting principles that will help you envision and enact a mutually supportive relationship. It is pictured in Figure 2.1. As you are read about these principles, think about what they mean to you.

Mutual Vulnerability

Mutual vulnerability means each of you approaches the other with a spirit of openness, curiosity, and self-honesty. You are willing to admit mistakes and feel safe to express your needs. Jason has

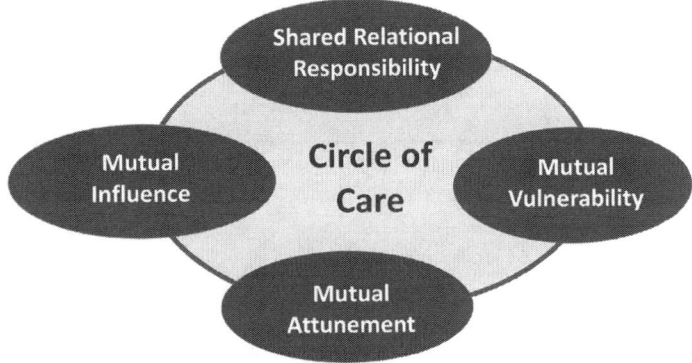

Figure 2.1 Orienting Principles for Mutually Supportive Relationships.

been socialized to not let himself be vulnerable. This makes it hard to be open to Rebecca's needs or acknowledge his need for her. As long as they did not venture into difficult terrain, he felt comfortable in the relationship. Over time, Rebecca learned not to raise disruptive subjects. Though each experienced vulnerabilities based on what they perceive is expected in their roles—Jason needs to appear competent, Rebecca needs to be a "good" mother—Rebecca was in a more vulnerable position because she could not express her needs without distressing Jason and was socialized to keep relationships smooth. Since learning to practice mutual vulnerability, Jason is more able to be in touch with and express his own relational needs and take in hers. This validates Rebecca and makes it easier for her to express her needs and dreams.

Check your mutual vulnerability

- ❑   Are you each willing to show weakness, uncertainty, or mistakes in your partner's presence?
- ❑   Do you each feel safe and willing to share your innermost thoughts and feelings with your partner?
- ❑   Are you each likely to seek relationship repair by expressing a feeling or concern?

Mutual Attunement

Mutual attunement means you each notice your partner's needs and are attentive and responsive to their experience. While learning to openly express yourself is valuable, you don't expect your partner to always have to tell you what is going on for them. You orient yourself to paying attention, to taking in their experience, and responding accordingly. Jason was quite good at attuning to their young children, but did not actively attune to Rebecca unless she was upset. And then he tried to "fix it" without really taking in what was going on for her. Rebecca tried to attune to everyone in the family, but hurt and resentment at not feeling "felt" often got in the way. Learning to orient toward each other, especially when they were struggling, was a major step toward a mutually supportive relationship.

Check your mutual attunement

- ❑   How interested are each of you in knowing and understanding your partner?
- ❑   Do you each listen to your partner? About what? In what circumstances?
- ❑   Do you each notice your partner's feelings and needs? Do you respond to them?

Mutual Influence

Mutual influence means you are each willing to accommodate and be changed by the other; that each of your needs and interests shape relationship patterns and choices. Without realizing it, Jason's needs and interests had been organizing their relationship. This is not what either partner wanted. Jason believed he was willing to be influenced by Rebecca and the children, but he needed to more intentionally orient toward their "we." Rebecca was worn out from trying to accommodate everyone in the family. Her rather automatic accommodation and attention to Jason—not in everything, but in many ways that went unnoticed—made it easier for Jason to assume everything was OK, or that Rebecca's problems were "hers." Once Jason saw what was happening, he was receptive to making changes. In turn, Rebecca felt safer to express her needs and interests, and more entitled to have them matter.

Check your mutual influence

- ❑   Can each of you engage your partner in addressing issues that concern you?
- ❑   Does each of you feel free to express opinions or make requests?
- ❑   Does each of you shift your interests/schedule to fit your partner's interests and schedule?

Shared Relational Responsibility

Shared relational responsibility means each of you does what is necessary to maintain the relationship. You each focus on the other as well as yourself and are accountable for your effect on your partner. Neither Jason or Rebecca believes that responsibility for their relationship should rest more on her shoulders than his. But because they did not talk about it, an imbalance in relational responsibility and care work evolved without conscious awareness. Once Jason sees how he is (unintentionally) impacting Rebecca, he immediately wants to make changes. Sometimes these changes pull up messages based on individualism and stereotypic masculinity that make him feel like he shouldn't accommodate, but awareness of his relational interests and values help him through. It is sometimes hard for Rebecca to let go of the expectation that responsibility for the relationship rests on her, but the more she and Jason talk and share responsibility for their relationship, the better she feels:

Check your shared relational responsibility:

- ❑ Do you each focus on what is needed to maintain or improve your relationship?
- ❑ Do each of you keep track of what needs to be done for the family? For your partner(s)?
- ❑ How responsible are each of you for doing the emotional work in the relationship?

Orienting Toward Relationship

Orienting toward relationship contradicts many societal messages regarding individualism, competition, achievement, and economic success. It does not mean you have to give up all your individuality or personal aspirations. It means that you and your partner(s) are able to address your needs, interests, and goals together. You approach challenges, crises, and opportunities through a foundation that holds and supports each of you and makes the relationship a priority.

> Rebecca and Jason have now been married for 23 years and are parenting young adults. Though parenting is a demanding time of life that tends to stress couple relationships, Jason and Rebecca learned to turn toward each other when problems arise. When they are angry, they recognize and appreciate that there are two voices in their relationship. They are even willing to be temporarily uncomfortable to take in each other's perspective and learn what is going on between them. They feel closer now than ever. When Rebecca was diagnosed with breast cancer four years ago, they were able to make the changes needed to accommodate the physical and emotional demands of cancer treatment, while still juggling parenting and work responsibilities. What mutual support looked like was different than before, but practicing the Circle of Care enabled the flexibility needed to respond to this crisis.

In the chapters that follow you will develop awareness of the socio-emotional influences that affect how you relate to one another and learn how to apply each principle of the Circle of Care to your unique circumstances and relational goals.

List at least two relational goals that are important to you:

_____

_____

_____

Conversation 2

This conversation will help you identify your relational values and experiences. If you are doing it with your partner, it is a way to open discussion about what mutual support will mean to each of you. Before beginning, take a moment to orient yourself relationally:

- Make yourself comfortable and close your eyes
- Be aware of your breath as it gently goes in and out
- Be aware of any tension, worry, or judgment. Gently let them go
- Picture yourself connected within a world of relationships
- Be aware of any tension, worry, or judgment. Gently let them go
- Open your eyes. Be aware of your conversational partner(s)
- Be aware of your desire to know them

This conversation follows the structure you used in the prior chapter. Each of you responds to the first question before moving on to the second and so on. Listeners do not interrupt or comment. When speaking, take time to let your thoughts evolve. Allow yourselves up to two minutes per question. Alternate who begins the next question. If you are doing the exercise without a partner, write your answers and then read them aloud to yourself. Hearing your own voice matters.

1   Share a story about a time when you needed someone. How did you respond? How did others respond? What is important to you about this story?

2   What societal messages regarding individuality (assertiveness, being "right," achievement, dominance, etc.) have been part of your life? Share examples of how they have affected you.

3   What societal messages regarding relationality (warmth, empathy, cooperation, accommodation, etc.) have been part of your life? Share examples of how they have affected you.

4   Share a story about a time your partner's (or intimate other's) care had a positive impact on you. Why is this important to you?

5   Share an area where you struggle or are confused regarding what it means to be relational. Where do you get stuck? What would you like to better understand?

6   As you listen to your conversational partner(s), what would like to learn more about? What would this mean to you? (Partners do not answer.)

7   As you listen to your conversational partner(s), what new awareness is evolving for you? How is this helpful to you?

Additional Resources

Commitment to mutual support. Copy the Circle of Care from Appendix B at the back of the book or download it by visiting www.routledge.com/9781032759890 and clicking on the link that says "Support Material." Post it where you can see it regularly. There is space at the bottom for each of you to state your commitment to mutual support in your own words. Use this as an opportunity to regularly remind yourselves of your commitment to mutuality and the Circle of Care.

Care work checklist. Use this checklist to raise your awareness of what is involved in the "care work" that typically remains invisible. You can download it (as above) or copy it from Appendix C at the back of this volume. Consider how this work is important and helpful, who does it, and how it can be shared more fairly.

Chapter 3

Develop Socio-Emotional Awareness

You have absorbed a lot of ideas about what is "normal" or "natural." What these are depends on the larger society, the nature of your family and community, how these ideas affected you, and how you responded. If you are like most people, you take these ideas for granted. They simply "are." Perhaps you have questioned, resisted, or reflected on some of them. Even if you are aware of or have witnessed a variety of societal standards and expectations, many sociocultural messages and their effect on you and your relationships almost certainly remain invisible.

Sociocultural ideas frame what you think, feel, and do. They affect how you judge yourself and others and how others view you. They guide how you relate and engage in the world. In this chapter you will begin to develop socio-emotional awareness that will help you recognize the impact of societal experiences in your life and increase the personal and relational possibilities available to you.

What is socio-emotional awareness?

- Sensitivity to the effect of cultural norms and expectations in your life
- Consideration of who has the power to define social standards
- Awareness of how your place in society connects to your emotions

Like any skill, developing socio-emotional awareness takes intentional focus and practice. It can be challenging at first, but after a while it becomes almost automatic. It will help you and your partner know yourselves better, avoid automatically falling into societal patterns, and be more intentional about how you relate.

Example

Nicole, a dental hygienist, and Tyler, a self-employed electrician, have been married for 12 years and have two sons in middle school. Between work, parenting, and family and friends, they are going, going, going most of the time. Neither feels very connected to the other anymore and both seem easily irritated. At the suggestion of a friend, they are setting aside time to complete this workbook together. They find themselves discussing things they have never talked about before.

Where Did You Learn What is Normal?

Pause for a moment. Notice your breath going in and out. Picture the community in which you grew up. What were the ethnic or racial backgrounds of most of the people? How much money did most people have? Was you family similar or different? Who was respected? Why? What mattered? How was gender expressed? We'll explore these questions in more detail later. For now, jot down some thoughts that come to mind:

DOI: 10.4324/9781003476528-3

What was considered normal in the eyes of most people?

_____

_____

_____

What was expected of a good person? A respected person? Did this depend on race, gender, or income?

_____

_____

_____

How did these ideas affect you?

_____

_____

_____

These questions may be hard to answer. Don't worry. Now that you've questioned the idea of "normal," you will begin to see its impact on you. New awareness will come through the activities that follow and while going about your day.

Looking at how Nicole and Tyler came to define "normal" will help you get some perspective. While both identify as Black, their experiences are quite different.

Nicole grew up in a predominately White, middle-class neighborhood where she learned that maintaining appearances is important—lawn is mowed, clothes are in fashion, you keep noise down. Her parents responded by fitting in and doing what was needed to be accepted and successful at their jobs. Nicole learned that her skin color meant what she did was visible, and since they were "different," their family needed to stick together. Tyler grew up in a low income, predominately Black community where "everyone looked out for each other." What mattered was honesty and collective survival. Individual achievement was less important; when Tyler did well in science and trained to be an electrician, the whole neighborhood celebrated and, if they could, contributed funds to launch his business.

What is Your Felt Identity?

It is common in Euro-American society to talk about your "self" or "personhood" as though it is inside you, something you were born with or developed on your own. But of course, you don't come to know who you are in isolation. As you interact with others and they respond, you come to see and know yourself. The extent to which you are aware of this identity-defining activity varies from person to person and from one time and place in your life to another.

As you can see from the example of Nicole and Tyler, what the color of your skin means depends on where you are—so does the meaning of achievement or what your gender or sexuality mean to you and others. You do not just absorb these things; your response is also important. Some experiences emotionally register in your body more than others. Together, all these—your circumstances in the larger world, family and community, and your personal responses—form your identity: who you experience yourself to be. In the language of Socio-Emotional Relationship Therapy (SERT), this is your felt identity.

What is felt identity?

Your felt identity is not just a name for what some people call your "social locations" (your race, ethnicity, gender, sexuality, age, abilities, etc.) or the roles you play (spouse, parent, employee, etc.). You may not have a word for your felt identities or realize which are significant to you. But your body knows. Your felt identity is at the heart of your emotional reactions and why you do what you do. When personal interactions challenge your felt identity, you are likely to defend or protect it. The good news is that while identities create a sense of personal stability, they also change over time and from setting to setting. When you become aware of your felt identities, you have more choice.

Given her experience of normal, Nicole's felt identity includes a strong sense that she must perform all her roles in her life well according to standards of the larger White society. She feels anxious if she or her family members "look bad," like she's representing her race. In their mixed-race community, she is viewed as "professional" and a responsible neighbor and parent. Consistent with his experience of normal, Tyler's felt identity is less oriented to fitting in with White society. He feels a strong sense of responsibility toward meeting the needs of his customers and to a large network of family and friends with whom he has close ties and likes to have fun. When he knows a customer is financially strapped, he is likely to reduce or "forget" the charge.

Disappointments and arguments between Nicole and Tyler usually connect to these felt identities. Each carries strong commitment to family, but Tyler has a wider view of who that includes. Nicole sometimes judges Tyler as "not responsible;" for example, when he doesn't collect "delinquent" payments or when he spends time having fun with friends rather than on upkeep of their house. Tyler sometimes views Nicole as "up tight" and resists her "nagging." In these moments, their "felt identities" do not understand each other.

As with Tyler and Nicole, awareness of the various aspects of your felt identities and how they show up in your emotions and relationships is an important step toward better communication and connection.

Your Place in the World and What you Feel and Do

The following activity explores the impact on you of various aspects of your felt identities—your unique place in the world. For each, list your identity, the societal messages you received, what feelings they bring up, and how you usually respond. There are no "right" answers. Trust your first thoughts. Then ask yourself "what else?" Thoughts may come more quickly for some areas than others. Those you haven't thought about before can be important. Give each topic your attention. It's OK to come back if you need more time. Use the example of Nataliya (below) to prompt your reflections.

Example

Nataliya (aged 33) ended a seven-year relationship with Daniel when she realized how much he "put down" and controlled her. About a year later she started going out with Barry (aged 40). Barry is divorced and shares custody of his two young children. He does not want more children and has had a vasectomy. Five months ago, Nataliya moved in with Barry and his children. She loves Barry but sometimes feels anxious regarding the future. She is completing this workbook with two friends to better understand what she wants and expects in a relationship.

Nataliya's answers are listed in italics. Write your answers below hers.

Your biological sex and gender identity *female*

What stereotypes and expectations did you receive from society about what is expected, good, and valued?
Be a mother, be nurturing and kind
Be pretty and supportive
Look after my parents and husband
Be nice, keep things smooth

When you think about yourself in relation to these expectations and -stereotypes what do you feel?
Guilty, inadequate, selfish
Loss—I want to be a mother
Resentment—then more guilt

How do these messages affect how you relate to others?
I feel guilty when Barry is upset. Like I've failed. I try to be understanding, but sometimes I just "explode." Then Barry thinks I'm unreasonable or immature. If I stay with Barry, I will never be a "real" mother.

Additional thoughts/notes? *I didn't realize that not being a mother makes me feel like I'm not a woman. Or that I feel guilty for not being "nice"—like women "should"*

Your race and ethnicity *white, Romanian*

What stereotypes and expectations did you receive from society about what is expected, good, and valued?
White—I'm acceptable, credible, "normal," respectable, should work toward my goals
Romanian—foreign, stoic, expect bad things and endure, don't' trust

When you think about yourself in relation to these expectations and stereotypes what do you feel?
Grateful and an impostor. I look White, but I don't feel White; I feel pressure to achieve. I feel less than, anxious to perform.

How do these messages affect how you relate to others?
I try to fit in and not rock the boat. I'm not sure who to trust, so I don't get close easily. I work hard to act normal and be accepted. Barry appreciates who I am—when he's unhappy, I doubt myself.

Additional thoughts/notes? *My life is easier because I'm White, but there's a lot of me I hide—I suppose because people might not understand or approve.*

Your economic and educational level. *BA in marketing. Good job. Middle class now (but parents fled Romania with nothing)*

What stereotypes and expectations did you receive from society about what is expected, good, and valued?	When you think about yourself in relation to these expectations and stereotypes what do you feel?	How do these messages affect how you relate to others?
Money is security. In America, people who work hard should be successful. My value is in my work.	*Pressure to "succeed." No matter what I do, it is not enough. Disappointed in myself for not doing better.*	*I stayed with Daniel because he was successful—had good job and was respected.*

Additional thoughts/notes? *My career is a big part of my identity. I think Barry understands that.*

Your sexual orientation *bi-sexual, in relationship with a heterosexual man—most people assume I'm hetero*

What stereotypes and expectations did you receive from society about what is expected, good, and valued?	When you think about yourself in relation to these expectations and stereotypes what do you feel?	How do these messages affect how you relate to others?
Straight is good. Gay is OK. Bi is weird. If I'm bi, I must not be a real woman.	*Misunderstood, lonely, different*	*There's usually no natural way to tell people I'm bi. So they don't know me. Daniel hated it about me. Barry says he's good with it, but...he doesn't "get" it. So I keep that part of me to myself.*

Additional thoughts/notes:

Your culture and religion *no religion, Romanian culture*

What stereotypes and expectations did you receive from/about these regarding what is expected, good, and valued?	When you think about yourself in relation to these expectations and stereotypes what do you feel?	How do these messages affect how you relate to others?
Be obedient, cautious, don't expect too much because things can change.	*I feel ashamed when I resist family or society's rules. The thought of change makes me nervous.*	*I tend to accept bad relationships (like with Daniel and at work) in order to maintain stability. I don't easily step "out of bounds."*

Additional thoughts/notes? *No wonder I stayed so long with Daniel! I don't know what I'm entitled to in a relationship. I'm looking forward to learning more about the Circle of Care!*

Your body and abilities. *I have ADHD*

What stereotypes and expectations did you receive from society about what is expected, good, and valued? *I should be able to multi-task (and look good!). I can overcome anything if I work hard enough.*	When you think about yourself in relation to these expectations and stereotypes what do you feel? *Defective. Hopeless—I'll never be good enough. And pride at how much I've accomplished anyway.*	How do these messages affect how you relate to others? *Barry wants me to be more organized at home. I feel like he is right, that I should be! I feel guilty but also hurt that he doesn't understand how hard it is for me.*

Additional thoughts/notes? *I can't slack off at work because I have ADHD. I'm so tired when I get home....*

Your family structure (single parent, married, cohabiting, polyamorous, multigenerational, etc.) *cohabiting step-parent*

What stereotypes and expectations did you receive from society about what is expected, good, and valued? *Not married and "step" are second class, not real or recognized.*	When you think about yourself in relation to these expectations and stereotypes what do you feel? *I want to be Barry's first love. I want to be recognized as a mother. I feel less than.*	How do these messages affect how you relate to others? *I know I'm being silly, selfish. I can't change this, but I want Barry to understand what I am giving up.*

Additional thoughts/notes? *I want to understand more about this. It's important to me.*

Your emigration experience and legal statuses *2nd generation. Parents immigrated before I was born*

What stereotypes and expectations did you receive from society about what is expected, good, and valued?
Don't complain, be grateful. Work hard to honor parents' sacrifice. Make money.

When you think about yourself in relation to these expectations and stereotypes what do you feel?
That my individual needs are not important. That I'm selfish to want more, lonely.

How do these messages affect how you relate to others?
I feel guilty to want anyone's attention. I feel lucky that a man like Barry loves me—and ashamed to complicate his life.

Additional thoughts/Notes? *My parents lost everything in Romania. Their life always seemed to be about making money. They don't show love—but now I'm thinking that's how they show love.*

Other aspects relevant to you (list) *I am a dancer*

What stereotypes and expectations did you receive from society about what is expected, good, and valued?
Be perfect, always do better, Not marketable, not productive.

When you think about yourself in relation to these expectations and stereotypes what do you feel?
Ashamed that I didn't have what it takes to stick with it.

How do these messages affect how you relate to others?
I love to dance, but it takes time away from Barry, his kids, work, and my parents. I feel resentful sometimes that they don't appreciate what it means to me.

Additional thoughts/notes? When I dance, I feel focused, that I'm being me. But it's an "extra"– it's hard to find a place for it in my world.

What is Your Unique Place in the World?

As Nataliya reflected on how all her felt social identities come together in her life, she noticed themes of loneliness, feeling different in ways people can't see or understand, and values around work, money, and stability. Her needs for love, acceptance, and mutual support are not validated in her place in society. She knew being a mother was important to her, but hadn't realized that being a step-mother felt second class. She also had not realized how much she had been affected by her immigrant parents' pursuit of economic stability (i.e., the "American Dream") or how guilty and ashamed she feels when she upsets Barry or wants more for herself.

Take a moment to review your responses to the previous activity. Reflect on how all the aspects of your place in the world interconnect in your life and in your relationships. How do they affect how you feel about yourself and others? Where do you feel known and not-known? How do they affect your expectations and what matters to you? Where do you experience the ability to influence your world and where you do not?

What themes come to mind?

_____

_____

_____

Which societal standards seem to have the most impact on you?

_____

_____

_____

Where do you think these societal standards come from? Who or what in society do they benefit?

_____

_____

_____

How do these societal messages affect what you expect of yourself and your partner?

_____

_____

_____

What values do these societal messages emphasize? How do these fit with your relational values? (You may want to check your responses in the last chapter.)

_____

_____

_____

Expand Your Awareness

Completing these exercises was a big job! It is an important step toward awareness of your unique place in the world and how it affects you and your relationships. This is always a work in progress. Plan to come back to add to—or change—your initial responses as your awareness evolves. The next two chapters on emotion and power will help.

Share Your Felt Experience

An important part of knowing yourself is sharing your experience with others interested in knowing you. New awareness is more likely to have staying power when you voice it and others take it in. This is especially true if you are sharing something emotionally meaningful to you. If you are doing the conversation that follows with your intimate partner, it is an opportunity to know each other better without attempting to solve a problem or make a decision. Before you begin, pause to make yourself comfortable and orient to each other with curiosity.

Orient with curiosity

- Make yourself comfortable and close your eyes
- Be aware of your breath as it gently goes in and out
- Be aware of any tension, worry, or judgment. Gently let them go
- Open your eyes. Be aware of your conversational partner(s)
- Be aware of your desire to know them

Conversation 3

This activity follows the basic conversational structure used in prior chapters. Each of you responds to the first question before moving on to the second and so on. Listeners do not interrupt or comment. When speaking, take time to let your thoughts evolve. Alternate who begins the next question. Following the structured format creates space for each of you to be heard. If you are doing the exercise without a partner, write your answers and then read them aloud to yourself.

1   Share a story that is meaningful to you regarding one aspect of your felt social identity (gender, race, economic status, sexuality, etc.). Why is it important to you today?

2   What moved you about your partner's story? How does hearing this story affect you?

3   Share a story that is meaningful to you regarding another aspect of your felt social identity (gender, race, economic status, sexuality, etc.). Why is it important to you today?

4   What moved you about your partner's story? How does hearing this story affect you?

5   Share a story that is meaningful to you regarding a third aspect of your felt social identity (gender, race, economic status, sexuality, etc.). Why is it important to you today?

6   What moved you about your partner's story? How does hearing this story affect you?

7   What new awareness, questions, or thoughts are stimulated for you by sharing these stories?

8   How does your experience of sharing these stories about your places in the world affect your awareness of how you relate to your partner and others?

Additional Resources

The Socio-Emotional Awareness Log. Use this as a way to journal or track your evolving socio-emotional awareness. You can copy it from Appendix D at the back of the book or download it by visiting www.routledge.com/9781032759890 and clicking on the link that says "Support Material." There are columns to note (a) what happened/what you felt, thought or did; (b) societal ideas related to your felt identities that were activated; and (c) how these affect your relationship/how you prefer to respond. You can start your reflections in either column.

For example, Nataliya was aware that she felt lucky that Barry loved her. She listed this in the first column, then she reflected on how these related to "less than" messages regarding her identity as a child of Romanian immigrants and feelings of inadequacy in how she fulfills her role as a woman, complicated by her experience with ADHD. In the final column, she noted that she held back from expressing her concerns to Barry and would prefer to feel worthy enough to speak her mind. Nataliya found that using the log helped her sort out her thoughts and get perspective.

Try the log and see if it works for you.

Chapter 4

Appreciate Emotion

Have you been told that you, or someone you know, are too emotional? Or that good leaders are not emotional? For generations, people have been taught that emotion gets in the way of rational thought; that emotions are "primitive" or dangerous—that if you show emotion, you risk not being taken seriously or judged less mature. In fact, just the opposite is true. Scientists now know that access to emotion is necessary to make good decisions. In his ground-breaking book, *Emotion, Reason, and the Human Brain* (1995), Antonio Damasio changed how neurobiologists understand the links between thinking and feeling; that if the part of your brain that processes emotion is damaged, you will not be able to think clearly, to make sound decisions. Evaluating information and responding appropriately requires emotional input.

This is not to say that the emotion underlying your thinking and judgments is always the most helpful read of the situation or that it is "unbiased." But if you are not aware of your emotions or your emotional functioning is restricted, your ability to effectively take in and respond to others and the world around you is limited. This chapter will help you appreciate emotion, how it connects you with your world, and why it is important to the changes you want to make.

Emotion Connects You with Your World

Like all humans, you are a social creature that adapts to your environment. Emotion connects your body with the world around you. It is always situational. Your emotional system reads how safe you are and your power position, and almost instantaneously tells you how to respond while communicating information about you to others. It is a relational experience.

Imagine yourself in an emotional situation. Pick an instance in which your sense is positive (love, joy, feeing valued, excited, happy, etc.). Look at Figure 4.1. Your positive feeling is at the center of an emotional moment in which you experience yourself in relation to your environment. It connects your body with what is happening around you. You intuit where power lies and how safe it is. What you think, feel, and do intertwine.

As you pause to reflect on this positive moment:

- Where do you feel this positivity in your body (your chest? your breathing? your gut? your shoulder and neck? your muscles?) What sensations do you feel?

- What thoughts come to mind about you and those around you?

- In this moment, what do cultural ideas say about you and those around you (what is good/not good, important, expected, right/wrong)?

DOI: 10.4324/9781003476528-4

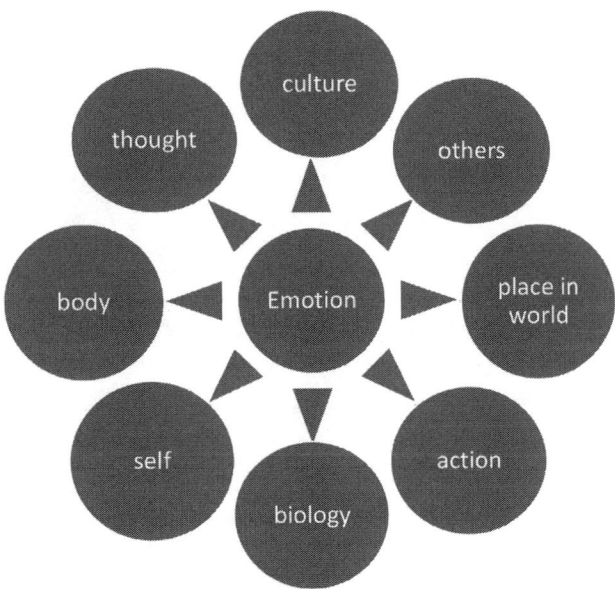

Figure 4.1 My emotional map.

- What does this moment tell you about your place in the world (your power position, how safe you are, your worth?)

Now think of an instance in which your emotional experience is negative (hurt, sadness, anger, fear, loneliness, etc.). Take a moment to consider what happens:

- Where do you feel this negativity in your body (your chest? your breathing? your gut? your shoulder and neck? your muscles?) What sensations do you feel?

- What thoughts come to mind about you and those around you?

- In this moment, what do cultural ideas (what is good/not good, important, expected, right/wrong) say about you and those around you?

- What does this moment tell you about your place in the world (your power position, how safe you are, your worth?)

You probably noticed that your body responded very differently to the positive emotional experience than the negative one. And the messages about yourself and your social situation are also different. How your body reacts depends on the social messages—the situational stories—that give meaning to what you experience. Let's look a little more closely at what happens.

The Socio-Emotional Circuit

When you experience an emotional event, many things happen in your body all at once. They are triggered as you interact with others and experience your place in the world—who you are in relation to others, how you are viewed, what is expected of you, and how you know yourself. As illustrated in Figure 4.2, when

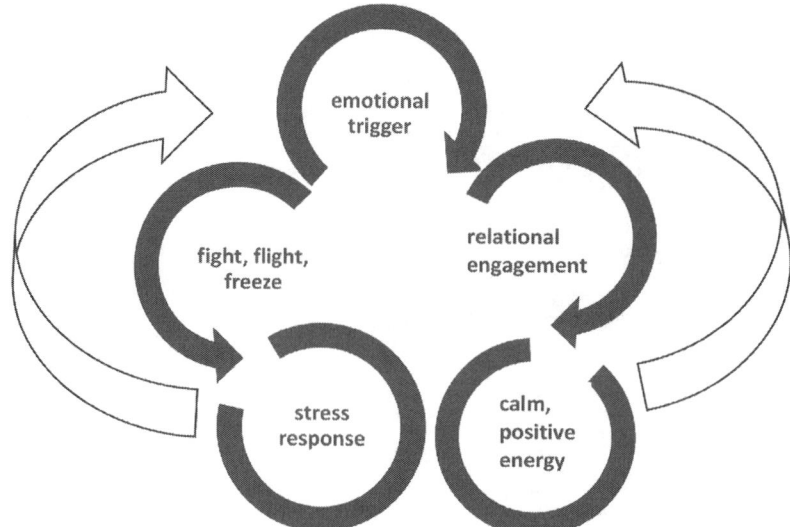

Figure 4.2 The Socio-Emotional Circuit.

your relational networks are safe, trustworthy, and supportive, they serve as a calming force and inspire positive energy. When they are not, you may protect yourself by fighting, shutting down, and/or disengaging. Your prior experiences and their ongoing effect on how your body responds to stress influence how you are likely to react now. At the same time, each emotional situation opens new possibilities.

To see how this socio-emotional circuit works, let's look at Dave and Miguel:

> *Miguel (38) and Dave (46) have been married for 12 years—since before same gender marriages were protected in all states. When they met, Miguel was closeted and had a called-off engagement with a woman and only brief flings with men. Dave, whose heritage is Anglo American, was part of an active gay community and had enjoyed a rich sexual life with a variety of partners. Dave had been out to his family for many years and maintained cordial, but distant relationships with them. Miguel was close to his Mexican American parents, extended family, and community. When Dave and Miguel met, their sense of connection was almost instantaneous. Miguel felt welcomed in Dave's gay community, but hid his relationship with Dave from his parents until they decided to marry. Miguel's parents reluctantly accepted their marriage, but implored Miguel to keep it secret from their friends and community. In recent years, communication between Dave and Miguel has become strained, especially when discussing the house Miguel inherited when his parents died.*

The Power of Positive Connection

As Dave and Miguel got to know each other, several things happened:

- Dave, who as a gay young man felt validated by his parents and the broader society only when he was successful on the soccer team and achieved well in school, learned to protect himself from relational hurt and disappointment by keeping others at an emotional distance. He was liked and respected in his family and friendship networks, but because he had to keep significant parts of himself outside these relationships, he did not experience the sense of emotional fittedness with others necessary for health and well-being. When he met Miguel, who seemed to reach inside to know him, oxytocin surged through this body. Known as the cuddle hormone, oxytocin helped smooth the way for him to feel more connected to Miguel and more able to feel trust, empathy, and generosity. Stress hormones such as cortisol—which always kept him a bit on edge—decreased, soothing him. He not only felt connected to Miguel, he felt energized and more open to new possibilities.

- Miguel, whose body suffered from a build-up of cortisol and other stress responses from needing to be on guard to protect his gay identity, also felt known in a way he never had before. This not only increased the flow of oxytocin in his body, he literally felt like he could breathe. Being able to participate in an openly gay community relaxed him and even lowered his blood pressure. He felt hopeful and optimistic for the future.

- Since marriage was not a taken-for-granted step for gay people at that time, Dave and Miguel discussed what it would mean to marry, how to support each of them despite inequities related to their racial differences and Dave's higher income and social connections. As a result of this commitment to mutuality, they felt valued and loved, and this helped each navigate their worlds. Their positive emotion was reflected in better physical and emotional health.

Pause to reflect on a moment when you felt positive connection with your partner.

How do you feel it in your body?

_____

_____

_____

_____

What feelings/thoughts about yourself and your place in the world are part of this moment?

_____

_____

_____

_____

The Pain of Negativity and Disconnection

Everyone experiences emotional pain sometimes. When you respond by moving toward others and these people provide a safe and welcoming place for you, your ability to respond positively is greater and the negative impact of the pain is less. Even when you are alone, thoughts of supportive people can soothe you. When fear or shame keep you from turning toward others, or safe and responsive others are not available, the other side of the socio-emotional circuit kicks in. This is when you may fight to defend yourself (and hurt others) or disconnect, fleeing relational connection through distance or distractions (affairs, alcohol/drugs, work, etc.). When no other options seem possible, you may freeze, disconnecting from everything. Depression or dissociation are ways your body can freeze.

Intimate partners inevitably hurt each other sometimes. Like Miguel and Dave, you may be both the primary source of support for each other and a periodic source of pain. Over time, some of the positive emotion that Dave and Miguel experienced with each other began to be interrupted by negative emotions that prompted disconnection and challenged their communication.

- When his mother died from a sudden heart attack, Miguel was grief-stricken. Dave tried to support Miguel by encouraging him to go for walks and bringing home their favorite foods. But Miguel was shut down and hard to reach. When Dave tried to "cheer him up," Miguel felt disconnected from him—Dave didn't seem to understand or appreciate his loss. Miguel's levels of serotonin—a neurochemical that regulates mood and other bodily functions—decreased. He experienced feelings of depression, a natural response to loss and disconnection.

- When Miguel turned inward and away from him, Dave felt abandoned and alone. Rather than recognize these feelings and what they said to him, Dave emotionally distanced from Miguel and increased his focus on work and other friends. His levels of oxytocin decreased and his cortisol levels increased, which negatively affected every organ of his body. Eventually Dave and Miguel returned to a regular pattern of activity with each other and their friends, but some of the connection between them was lost.

- When Miguel's father died of advanced pancreatic cancer a few years later, he inherited his parents' modest home in the Mexican American neighborhood in which he grew up. Miguel suggested he and Dave move there. Dave thought this was a bad idea. Whenever they tried to talk about it, their conversation almost immediately escalated into anger and hurt.

What can you learn from Dave and Miguel?

- Turning toward welcoming others is good for your health
- Emotional disconnection hurts you physically and relationally
- Emotion carries important information about you and your world

Emotion Tells You What's Important

Perhaps you learned to "power through" no matter what you are feeling—or to be disappointed in yourself or others for feeling down or upset. Maybe you direct anger toward others to avoid feeling bad about yourself. If your feelings are hurtful or uncomfortable, you probably try to make them go away or distract yourself. And like Miguel and Dave, there may be topics that seem too emotional to discuss.

The answer is simple: *listen to what emotion has to say.* But little in our society encourages you to appreciate your emotion or that of others. This is especially true for painful emotions, but it is also true for positive ones. In our fast-paced society, the message is "move on, get things done." We learn to look for quick fixes or a pharmacological solution.

Think of emotion as feedback from and about your environment—about the people and world around you. You need to be in touch with this input and use it. Develop the habit of simply stopping to notice and take in what you are experiencing.

Exercise

Pause. Notice your breath as it goes in and out. Reflect on your day.

Notice and describe three emotions you experienced.

_____

_____

_____

_____

_____

What messages about your social environment did you take in?

_____

_____

_____

_____

_____

How did you respond?

Who noticed?

Emotion communicates. It is important to also notice and take in what your partner is experiencing.

Exercise

Reflect on what you observed about your partner today. Notice and describe three messages you received regarding their emotional state.

How did you respond?

_____

_____

_____

_____

_____

How did your response affect your partner?

_____

_____

_____

_____

_____

Emotional Mapping

When you and your partner are fighting—or avoiding each other to avoid confrontation, emotional mapping will help you get to the bottom of what is really going on and what you need or want (see Figure 4.1, *My emotional map*, at the beginning of this chapter). You can print a copy of this worksheet from Appendix E at the back of the book or download it by visiting www.routledge. com/9781032759890 and clicking on the link that says "Support Material." Though you can begin the emotional map anywhere, one of the following usually works best:

- Begin with a focus on the sensations in your body, then move to each of the other circles on the map; OR
- Begin with the thoughts you are having (especially "shoulds" and "oughts"), then move to each of the other circles on the map

You don't need to address the circles in order, but make notes for each of them. Allow yourself time to feel and reflect. What you name the emotion at the center may change as your awareness increases.

Let's use Dave and Miguel's emotion around whether to move into the house Miguel inherited as an example. Their arguments get stuck on whether the move is "a good idea." Included in their emotional maps are personal, cultural, and physiological messages about each of them and what is important or needs to be protected. Awareness of these will help Dave and Miguel use the conflict as a way to know each other better—to build emotional connection, rather than disconnection. They can learn from emotion to help center their relationship while making the decision about where to live.

Miguel's Emotional Map

- *Where in my body am I responding?* When Dave says moving into my family home is a "bad idea," my gut clenches. I have trouble breathing. I feel my whole body closing off from Dave.
- *What thoughts am I having?* My first thought is that Dave doesn't care about me. My second thought is that Dave is embarrassed by my Mexican American background and neighborhood. I remember how much my parents loved me and feel bad that I disappointed them.
- *What cultural messages am I receiving?* I am less than. As an Anglo, Dave is "better" than me. As a Latino man I should honor and protect my parents. As my partner, Dave should value by culture and family.
- *What ideas about/from others are involved?* Their home was everything to my parents, their sign of success and stability. My Mexican American community doesn't respect me and my relationship with Dave. I want to be "out" in my community. I worry that Dave doesn't love me for who I "really" am.

- *What is my place in the world?* I have always been on the outside looking in. I didn't fit anywhere. My parents' house was a safe place, even when they did not know all of me.
- *What am I pushed to do?* I am pushed to honor my parents and their sacrifices for me. Selling their home would be disloyal. I am also pushed to want Dave to "sacrifice" for me—to do something because it matters to me.
- *What is happening biologically?* My stress level has been high since my parents died. There is so much to do as their heir and executor. My cortisol levels are probably high and my blood pressure is up. I am so tired, worn out.
- *What does this say about me?* An interesting question. I think it means I loved my parents and have mixed feelings about hurting them by marrying Dave. I want to feel more pride in who I am, and I'm not ready to let go of the safe place this home represents to me.
- *Name the emotion.* Under my anger and hurt—fear that I was a disloyal son and loss of my Mexican American identity.

As Miguel walked though his emotional map, he began to be aware of parts of his emotional experience he had thought were in the past. He began to have a clearer picture of how he sees himself and his world, and how Dave and the loss of his parents and Mexican American community are connected to his family home. He is more able to reflect on what matters to him on this issue.

Dave's Emotional Map

- *What thoughts am I having?* I keep thinking that Miguel is cut off from reality. His parents' house is not in a good neighborhood. We can afford something much better. We should sell the house and invest the money in something that will appreciate more in value. Why does Miguel dismiss my input on this? Real estate is something I know a lot about.
- *Where in my body am I responding?* When Miguel dismisses my advice, my chest gets tight. My breathing gets faster and heavier. I feel pressure across my temples.
- *What cultural messages am I receiving?* As a successful man, I should know what I am talking about. Miguel should respect my knowledge about money and houses.
- *What ideas about/from others are involved?* Where we live reflects on our respectability as a couple. I have worked so hard to be successful and get people's respect. I don't want to be known as "the gay couple" in a community that judges me.
- *What is my place in the world?* Miguel and I have a good life in a good community and lots of friends that appreciate and value me. I have accomplished a lot—my "standing" is good. Why would I risk that, especially in a place where I don't fit in?
- *What am I pushed to do?* I feel pushed to make Miguel understand why I am right and take my advice. I also feel pushed to defend myself—that I'm not a racist or bigot.
- *What is happening biologically?* I'm sure my blood pressure goes up around this issue. I feel my heart shutting down when Miguel and I fight.
- *What does this say about me?* Hmmm. I guess it's important to be respected. If Miguel doesn't listen to me, he must not respect me. Maybe I'm not really important to him—not really his family.
- *Name the emotion.* Under my anger is fear that I'm not worthy, that Miguel doesn't respect me. How can he love someone he doesn't respect?

Walking through his emotional map helped Dave be aware of his lifelong vulnerability around needing to be recognized as "successful." Because he always presents such a confident image, it was helpful to become aware of his hidden worry that he is not good enough to be loved.

Sharing Socio-Emotional Awareness

Once Miguel and Dave were aware of their emotional maps, they had more choice about how to respond to their conflict. They realized that they were not arguing about the house, so much as about their felt identities. They needed to turn toward each other to address the complexity of Miguel's loss of his parents and Mexican American identity and how to bring his gay identity and family/cultural identity together. Sharing their emotional maps also made Dave's need for belonging and acceptance visible—something he had kept hidden from Miguel and even from himself. Whatever they decide about where to live and what to do with the house, mapping their emotion brought them closer together and better able to support each other through loss and change.

Sharing your evolving socio-emotional awareness with each other increases your emotional connection and helps you center your relationship as you make decisions and address conflict. This awareness will help you:

- Recognize and appreciate what is important to you
- See how what you feel connects to your relationships and place in the world
- Use this awareness to improve your relational connections

Conversation 4

This conversation is an opportunity to give voice to the messages you learned about emotion. Talking about it helps you begin to develop your own story about emotion and how to appreciate it in your life. If you are doing this conversation with your intimate partner, it is an opportunity to focus on each of your experiences around emotion without a problem you need to resolve.

Orient with curiosity

- Make yourself comfortable and close your eyes
- Be aware of your breath as it gently goes in and out
- Be aware of any tension, worry, or judgment. Gently let them go
- Open your eyes. Be aware of your conversational partner(s)
- Be aware of the larger world connected to each of you
- Be aware of any tension, worry, or judgment. Gently let them go
- Be aware of your interest in knowing your partner(s)

This activity follows the basic conversational structure used in prior chapters. Each of you responds to the first question for up to two minutes before moving on to the second and so on. Listeners do not interrupt or comment. When speaking, take time to let your thoughts evolve. Alternate who begins the next question. Following the structured format creates space for each of you to be heard. If you are doing the exercise without a partner, write your answers and then read them aloud to yourself.

1   Share a story that illustrates a societal message you received about emotion. Why is it important to you now?

2   Share a story about how others responded to your emotion? How did this affect you?

3   Share a story that shows how you learned to notice and respond to the emotion of others (or not). How has this affected your relationships?

4   As you've been listening to your conversational partner's stories about emotion, what has moved you? How? What would you like your partner to know?

5   As you've been reflecting on your conversational partner's stories about emotion, what new ideas, thoughts, or questions come up for you? What would you like to know more about? (Partner does not answer.)

6   As you reflect on this conversation, what new awareness and/or commitment do you bring to your relationship with your partner? What will this new awareness and/or commitment say about you and your relationship?

Additional Resources

My emotional map. You can make copies of "My emotional map" from Appendix E at the back of the book or download it by visiting www.routledge.com/9781032759890 and clicking on the link that says "Support Material." When faced with an emotionally challenging situation, use this map to increase your personal emotional awareness of what is happening for you. Begin with your bodily sensations and emotional state and move outward toward the other circles. The map includes questions to help you reflect on what this emotion says about what is important to you and what it means in your relationships and place in the world.

My partner's emotional map. You can make copies of "My partner's emotional map" from Appendix F at the back of the book or download it by visiting www.routledge.com/9781032759890 and clicking on the link that says "Support Material." Use this to imagine what your partner's emotional map may be in a particular situation. Begin with the outer circles and move toward likely emotion, thoughts, and bodily responses. The map includes questions to help you consider what may be important to your partner in this situation and what you are curious to know more about.

Chapter 5

Explore the Flow of Power

Power is your ability to have an impact on your world—to have what you say and feel respected, valued, understood, and viewed as credible, and for others to be open to your influence. In a mutually supportive relationship, power flows back and forth between you and your partner relatively equally. For example, each of you:

❑ Automatically imagines and considers your partner's feelings and needs
❑ Is able to freely express what concerns you
❑ Listens to and remembers what your partner says
❑ Takes your partner's concerns seriously
❑ Takes the other into account when making decisions
❑ Willingly makes changes to accommodate your partner and the family
❑ Remembers the details of the other's life
❑ Is attentive to what needs to be done in the household

These relational actions sound reasonable, don't they? If you love each other, mutual power should be easy. But it's not.

Even though most of us don't like to think about power, especially when we're in love, the workings of power are part of any relationship. In this chapter you will explore how power flows between you and your partner. You will learn that good intentions are not enough. Loving each other is not enough. The messages you receive from the outside world, how people treat you, and what that feels like all play a part in how you interact. Once you see how power flows between you, you can be accountable for your impact on the other. You can develop more equitable ways of relating.

Pause. Take a few breaths.
What comes up for you as you contemplate thinking about power between you and your partner(s)?

_____

_____

_____

_____

_____

DOI: 10.4324/9781003476528-5

Charting New Territory

If thinking about power in your relationship makes you anxious—or angry, or on guard—you are not alone. In *Marriage, a History: From Obedience to Intimacy, How Love Conquered Marriage*, family historian Stephanie Coontz (2005) explained that in the 21st century, you are charting new territory:

> For thousands of years marriage was organized in ways that reinforced female subservience ... today we have all inherited unconscious habits and emotional expectations that perpetuate female disadvantage in marriage.
>
> (p. 311)

The old rules were based on a power difference between men and women. Men controlled all the resources and were expected to keep their wives "in line." Those who could not were ridiculed. Women were taught to "play dumb" and become skilled in knowing how to accommodate and please their mates.

Times have changed. Today, women are increasingly unwilling to stay in relationships with unequal power. And many men are now attracted to strong, competent women. Men—not just women—do better in when power is equitable. But old habits and expectations based on inequality persist. If you are like most of us, you fall short of your egalitarian ideals. This is especially true if your partner's gender is different than yours.

The gendered nature of power influences which of you develops competencies in housework and child care, who automatically juggles work and family obligations, and who attends to family schedules and social connections. It continues old habits and patterns ways of relating that reinforce male dominance even when you don't intend it.

History teaches men they are entitled to dominate. Writing to couples, Ken Dolan-Del Vecchio (2008) offered these examples of how modern men perpetuate their power, usually without realizing you are doing so:

- ❑ Unselfconsciously prioritizing your own feelings and desires over those of your partner and other family members
- ❑ Making decisions on behalf of others without consulting them
- ❑ Forgetting about your partner's distress, feelings, or schedules even when they were expressed recently

History also teaches women to behave in ways that support male dominance. For example:

- ❑ To let men pass as more intelligent, skilled, or important
- ❑ To avoid direct disagreement with your partner and say things in a way that will not upset him
- ❑ To anticipate what your partner wants and focus on the things that interest him

Naming these old rules makes their anti-relational nature stand out. You probably don't agree with them. Yet most of us enact them in more ways than we realize. This lack of awareness is especially true when the relational flow puts you in a power position.

Power is Relational

How can you hold power if you do not intend it? How can you end up in a subservient position when you don't see yourself as "less than?" It is because power, as we are thinking of it here, is not a personal capacity within you; it is the result of an interpersonal process *between* people. Those who end up in a power position have more capacity to influence their partners and relationships. The one-down partner(s) contributes as well, willingly or unwillingly; however, responsibility for change cannot rest primarily with less powerful partners. It will not work, is not fair, and is often harmful (depression, resentment, etc.).

The old model of power is based on a hierarchy; one person (or group) has *power over* another person or group. My colleague Mona Fishbane (2013) teaches couples to practice *power with*, to work as a team to "cultivate equality, mutuality, and respect" through commitment to the well-being of each partner and to the relationship. She says this requires you counteract "cultural and neurobiological forces that lead to reactivity, self-protection, and power struggles" (p. 165). You learn to respond differently than what your mind and body have absorbed from the larger society. This takes intentionality and practice.

Shared power is not just a good idea. It is essential to couple success. For example, John Gottman's (2011) research can reliably predict which relationships will succeed and which will fail. Among successful couples, each partner is willing to be influenced by the other. It is not enough to expect your partners to always tell you nicely what they need; you need to also be open to influence from your partner's *negative* expressions (such as anger or hurt). Gender stereotypes tell women to do this, but encourage men to resist. Successful couples counteract these gender stereotypes and share power. This creates a foundation of safety and trust:

> Mistrust and betrayal are more likely to occur in marriages in which the husband has more power than the wife ... and in which she does not have very much power to influence him with her negativity.
>
> (Gottman, p. 432)

If you are like most modern couples, you want to share power. But seeing how power works between you can be tricky. This is because:

✓ Power is hidden in social norms and expectations
✓ If you're in a position of power, power is hard to see
✓ You may hold power, but not feel powerful

Exploring the flow of power in your relationship requires honest questioning and reflection to see what most of us are socialized not to see—particularly if you are in a position of power that is invisible to you. Naming power makes it possible to address it.

What models about the flow of power have been part of your life? From who?

_____

_____

_____

_____

What did these models say about your place in your family? In your community? In society?

_____

_____

_____

_____

_____

What did these models say about who you are and what you should do?

_____

_____

_____

_____

_____

Sources of Power

Power imbalances occur among all kinds of couples. Gender is a primary source of power in society. It intertwines with other sources of power to shape couple communication and intimacy. Consider which of the following sources of social power you and your partner(s) bring to your relationships. Most likely, you have both sources of power and sources of disadvantage. It is also likely that you and your partner do not enter the relationship with the same levels of social power.

❑ Gender
❑ Race and ethnicity
❑ Skin color
❑ Social class background
❑ Access to money
❑ Level of education and type of job
❑ Sexual orientation and preferences
❑ Abilities and how they are/are not valued
❑ Looks and how they fit dominant culture standards of attractiveness
❑ Country of origin, language you speak, and legal status
❑ Religious affiliation, including whether dominant or marginalized in society
❑ Size and physical strength
❑ Health and mobility
❑ Age and how it is viewed in society

As you reflect on this list, which of your characteristics carry social power?

_____

_____

_____

_____

_____

Which are sources of disadvantage?

_____

_____

_____

_____

_____

How do they compare with your partner's sources of power and disadvantage?

_____

_____

_____

_____

Sources of power like those listed above carry with them attitudes, expectations, and emotional experience. These are tied to how you feel about yourself and what you expect from others. Take a moment to reflect on what it feels like when you matter (a sign of power) and when you don't.

Think of an instance in your workplace or community where your voice and experience mattered. How did you feel? How did you respond?

_____

_____

_____

_____

Think of an instance in your workplace or community where your voice and experience were excluded or not understood. How did you feel? How did you respond?

_____

_____

_____

_____

Think of an instance in your relationship where your voice and experience mattered. How did you feel? How did you respond?

_____

_____

_____

_____

_____

Think of an instance in your relationship where your voice and experience were excluded or not understood. How did you feel? How did you respond?

_____

_____

_____

_____

_____

How Does Power Flow in Your Relationship?

When power is balanced each of you feels cared about, valued, and respected and you are equally able to influence the relationship and each other. To explore how power flows in your relationship consider seven questions:

1   Who is focused on the other and on maintaining the relationship?
2   Whose needs and interests are centered?
3   Whose voice matters?
4   Who is willing to accommodate?
5   How are conflict and decisions managed?
6   Who has choice regarding what household and childcare tasks you do?
7   Whose health and well-being are benefitted by the relationship?

As you ask these questions about your own relationship, use Bobbi and Armand as an example to stimulate your thoughts.

Bobbie (age 42) and Armand (age 49) are a White heterosexual couple married for 14 years. It is a second marriage for Armand. They have three children ages 10, 12, and 18 (oldest is Bobbi's daughter from a prior relationship). Armand owns a real estate business; Bobbi is a stay-at-home mom. They are completing this workbook at the suggestion of their therapist, whom they are seeing regarding conflicts about raising the children, money, and managing the household. They also had counseling four years ago after Bobbie had a brief affair. When angry, both are likely to verbally lash out. Bobbie usually leaves these encounters drained of energy and feeling guilty for her behavior, while Armand feels emotionally activated and irritated that his peace has been disturbed.

When they looked at their sources of social power, Bobbie and Armand identified that:

a   Both were socialized according to old gender rules; Armand learned he should be in charge and accommodated; Bobbie learned not to expect men to attune to her, that only her body was important.

b   Both take the benefits of whiteness for granted. When he was younger, Armand was ashamed because his French Canadian parents did not live up to the standards of the larger Anglo community.

c   Both were raised in "poor" neighborhoods. When Bobbie was a single mother, she had little money.

d   Armand makes a good income, which they view as a sign of success.

e   Armand worked hard to obtain a college degree and acceptance in the community; Bobbie graduated from high school despite little family support.

f   Before marrying Armand, Bobbie worked as a model. Armand sees having an attractive wife as a sign of his success.

g   Bobbie is depressed (low energy, hopelessness, despair).

Going through the list of power sources helped Armand realize that as a White heterosexual male with a college degree and good income, he brings more socially based power to the relationship than Bobbie. Both realized that Armand's financial success is important to their sense of value in the world, and Bobbie feels grateful that his income enables her to be a stay-at-home mom—a status she had thought was out of reach for her.

Who is Focused on the Other and on the Relationship?

As Armand reflects on when and how he focuses on Bobbie, he at first thinks he focuses on her a lot. He feels responsible for the family and wants her to be happy. And he wants her approval and respect. But as he looks closer, Armand realizes that he never learned how to see Bobbie for herself, rather than a reflection of him. He likes to see her smile, but does not often notice what is going on for her emotionally or stop to put himself in her place. Thinking about it now, Armand *does* want to know what Bobbie is thinking and feeling, but he is not in the habit of focusing on her; he's not sure he knows how (see Chapter 7).

Bobbi is aware that she regularly monitors how Armand is feeling and what he wants. She realizes she was taught that it is her job to soothe him and make him feel good, to take care of their relationship. Now that she is looking at the patterns between them, she realizes that she often hides what she is feeling and thinking from Armand. She does not want to upset him and she does not believe he is interested. She can think of times when she did share something important and he did not understand or forgot. Taking stock now, she is aware that she carries resentment about his inattentiveness, and though she usually lets it go in appreciation of all Armand does give her, sometimes she erupts in anger or shuts down in hurt. Their difference in who focuses on the other creates a power imbalance.

Whose Needs and Interests are Centered?

Bobbie is aware that she learned to put Armand and the children's needs and interests first. She usually takes a lot of satisfaction in seeing them all do well. She has a family and economic security, and these are what matter most to her. Until they discussed it, Armand was not aware of how much his schedule and interests organized their life. It seemed natural to him. He also had not realized how much his interests in work and moving to a bigger and better house, joining the country club, and looking good in the community were measures of success imposed by his attachment to dominant culture expectations that matter less to Bobbie.

Bobbie and Armand discover a power imbalance that centers his interests and aspirations while reinforcing socio-economic standards that frequently take priority over their relational values. Another imbalance is harder to see. Armand loves to do things for Bobbie; he wants to make her happy. But he is in the habit of planning or buying something without first knowing what really matters to her. Bobbie appreciates the gestures, but does not feel felt by him.

Whose Voice Matters?

Bobbie often spends considerable time debating whether to raise a topic that matters to her, and when and how to do it. She knows that if she approaches him "right," Armand is more likely to listen and take her seriously. If she doesn't, Armand often dismisses her concerns as not important, unrealistic, or an affront to him. Learning the power of his voice is a surprise to Armand. He usually says what he wants, when he wants, without thinking about it. As he thinks about it now, he sees that when he thinks her topic is not important or will be upsetting, he often avoids discussion. He also realizes that he *does* want Bobbie's voice to matter.

Bobbie and Armand discover they have fallen into a common pattern they do not want: Armand determines which topics are important. Their arguments are an exception—a power struggle over whose voice matters. These conflicts happen when Bobbie cares enough about an issue to persist or when resentments that have been held back simply erupt. Their arguments are actually a sign that there are still two voices in their relationship.

Who is Willing to Accommodate?

Bobbie and Armand know making a life together takes mutual accommodation. They have a hard time seeing how this works between them until they ask themselves what it is like when they accommodate. Armand notices that when he accommodates to something Bobbie wants or is doing, he often feels like he is "giving in." He feels pulled—he wants to cooperate, but he feels "controlled" or "weak" when he does. He sees how the old rule that he should be in charge affects him, and realizes that he doesn't accommodate as often, or as comfortably, as he thinks he does.

Bobbie notices she often automatically accommodates; that as she plans her day or routine, she thinks about Armand's schedule and his needs and preferences, and organizes around that. Until they name it, neither she or Armand realize how much she accommodates—it just seems natural. The old rule that women should be flexible and not question keeps things smooth. When she asserts herself, she often feels selfish or guilty—or wonders if she expecting "too much." The imbalance in who accommodates limits conflict, but also limits flexibility and the degree to which Bobbie's interests and well-being are supported.

How are Conflict and Decisions Managed?

Armand and Bobbie agree on a lot of things. They share most life values. When conflict arises, it is usually because one person's preferences or expectations about raising children or how orderly to keep the house are not being met. Bobbie used to accommodate Armand on many of these issues, but recently is less willing to do so. Sometimes her resistance comes out as attack and anger. When this happens, Armand uses slurs and insults regarding Bobbie's previous affair like a club, which triggers Bobbie's guilt and leaves her speechless.

Armand and Bobbie begin to see their responses to conflict in light of the flow of power between them. They discover that the affair temporarily shifted the power imbalance in which Armand was not focused on what Bobbie feels and needs. The affair made Armand feel the vulnerability of his otherwise unacknowledged need for her and ashamed of his reduced power position—a violation of the old rule that he should be in control and not feel or show weakness. Though the affair felt good to Bobbie in the moment, she felt tremendously guilty and, after confessing, increased her efforts to tend and soothe Armand, which reinforced the old power imbalance. Now, when Bobbie's anger begins to again shift the flow of power, Armand's attacks about the prior affair shift the power back to him, but leave them disconnected from each other and unable to address their differences.

A note about affairs

The meaning of an affair may differ depending on the flow of power. When, like Bobbie, it is committed by a person in a one-down position the affair is likely, in part, an attempt to compensate for the effects of powerlessness. When an affair comes from a position of entitlement it is more likely a symptom power, such as the old gender rules that allow men to take what they want or a reflection of some other source of power.

Who has Choice Regarding Household and Childcare Tasks?

Bobbie always wanted to be a stay-at-home mom. She was attracted to Armand, in part, because he offered a strong and stable presence and appeared to like the idea of providing for a family. He was also kind to her young daughter. Bobbie is delighted that Armand likes to do things with the children and takes an interest in their sports activities. Since he views his own father as "harsh" and "disinterested," Armand wants to be a "fun" dad. He also likes to cook. Given that the old rules put all the household and childcare tasks on women, Bobbie feels grateful for Armand's domestic contributions, which adds to their power imbalance.

As Bobbie and Armand look at the question of who has choice regarding household and childcare tasks, they see some complexity. Armand would be okay if Bobbie wanted a job outside the home; in fact, he'd welcome it. However, Armand does only those domestic chores he chooses (cooking) and leaves the less fun aspects to Bobbie. They have never discussed who will do what around the house or how to share parenting. Armand feels entitled to a more orderly home. Bobbie wants him to be more understanding of her workload and to back up her discipline of the children. Their arguments about the children and house open the possibility of a shift in power, one that may include more balance in who is emotionally grateful, as well as who does what.

Whose Health and Well-Being are Benefitted?

Bobbie and Armand discover that without intending it, there is a power imbalance that disadvantages Bobbie's emotional well-being. This is because the ability to be felt—to be understood, respected, and valued—and to have an influence on Armand and their relationship is less accessible to her. Bobbie's depressive symptoms are a symptom of this power imbalance; so is the unresolvable conflict between them. They now see Bobbie's earlier affair as an unhelpful response to the power imbalance.

The conflict and growing distance between Bobbie and Armand are distressing to both of them and put their marriage at risk. They need guidance for how to relate according to new rules based on mutual support. Each will do better as they learn to apply the Circle of Care. They will have more choice and flexibility about how they want to relate and parent, and will be better equipped to handle stresses in the outside world and to responsively face whatever life challenges are ahead of them.

A note about money

Bobbi is financially dependent on Armand, which adds to the imbalance of power in their relationship. However, research shows that most of these old gender patterns still happen when each partner works outside the home. Veronica Tichenor (2005) studied couples in which women made more money than their male partners. She concluded that these women:

> often work to bolster their husbands' masculinity by deferring to them … and avoiding displays of power. This can entail tremendous psychic costs for women as they monitor their behavior and sensor themselves to avoid looking too powerful.

(p. 185)

As you explore power in your relationship—and how it compares to Bobbi and Armand—what are your first thoughts and impressions?

_____

_____

_____

_____

_____

Do you notice any gaps between the mutuality you seek and what actually happens in your relationship?

_____

_____

_____

_____

_____

How are you affected by the old rules that promote male dominance and female subservience?

_____

_____

_____

_____

_____

How might your partner be affected by these old rules?

_____

_____

_____

_____

_____

Developing Your Own Rules

This chapter has probably raised some thoughts that are new to you. Or perhaps it has given words to what you have known all along. Power can be challenging to see at first, but once you begin to see it—and if you are open to it—new opportunities arise. The flow of power between you and your partner is deeply personal; but it is influenced by power imbalances in the larger society and the power of the old rules. These old rules work against the relationships you want. The chapters that follow will help you develop new rules and create a fairer, more loving relationship that supports each of you.

Conversation 5

This conversation will help you bring the effect of power into the open. It is an opportunity to discuss power through an activity structured to make space for each of your voices. Whether with others or with your partner, the guidelines offer a safe and welcoming format for a conversation that may be new to you. As you begin, orient to your conversational partner(s) with curiosity and openness to learning.

Orient with curiosity

- Make yourself comfortable and close your eyes
- Be aware of your breath as it gently goes in and out
- Be aware of any tension, worry, or judgment. Gently let them go
- Open your eyes. Be aware of your conversational partner(s)
- Be aware of the larger world connected to each of you
- Be aware of any tension, worry, or judgment. Gently let them go
- Be aware of your interest in knowing your partner(s)

This activity follows the same conversational structure used in the previous chapters. Each of you responds to the first question for up to two minutes; then you move on to the second and so on. Listeners do not interrupt or comment. When speaking, take time to let your thoughts evolve. Alternate who begins the next question. If you are doing the exercise without a partner, write your answers and then read them aloud to yourself. It is important to hear your voice.

1   Share a story of a time when you felt respected and valued, that the other person(s) was interested in you. What did they do that told you that you matter? What was meaningful to you about this experience?

2   Share a story of a time when you felt less than, that who you are and what matters to you had little influence. What did the other person(s) do that told you that your experience or interests counted for little?

3   As you've been reading about power in this chapter, what ideas or thoughts were meaningful to you? Why are they important to you? Share an example.

4   When you consider the influence of old gender rules on modern relationships, what awareness about your own behavior and emotions comes to mind? Share an example. Why is this example important to you?

5   As you think about power and listen to your partner(s) in this conversation, what new questions come to mind? What are you uncertain about?

6   As you listened to your partner(s) in this conversation, what has moved you? What new awareness or insight have you gained? How are these important to you?

7   As you leave this conversation, what commitment are you making to yourself? To your partner? What is the potential impact of these commitments on the future?

Additional Resources

Your relational orientations. You can copy Appendix G from the back of the book or download it by visiting www.routledge.com/9781032759890 and clicking on the link that says "Support Material." It shows four general ways you can orient to power and relationships. Use these to explore the way you usually orient to relationships, a possible gap between the way you orient and the way you want to orient, and how you may orient differently to power and relational focus depending on the circumstances. You can also compare your relational orientation with your partner and discuss the type you prefer.

Undoing gendered power. Patriarchy is both a mindset and the way relationships and organizations are organized in society. As we've seen in this chapter, male dominance persists even when you want to be equal. Appendix H offers a list of patriarchal rules for men and boys that impact everyone (male, female, queer, nonbinary). You can download and/or print it to explore how you have been impacted by each rule and suggest a new rule to replace it.

Chapter 6

Express Mutual Vulnerability

Relationships are good for your health—and almost inevitably include emotional risks. How you and your partner respond to them makes all the difference. When you approach each other with a spirit of vulnerability, good communication and intimacy are possible; you will each feel safe to be open to the other. Mutual vulnerability is thus the first element of the Circle of Care (see Figure 6.1). This chapter will help you explore what is involved in mutual vulnerability and what it means to you. You will discover how mutual vulnerability creates a foundation of relational trust and take steps to enhance it in your life.

What is Vulnerability, and Why is It Important?

Relationships always involve uncertainties and potential areas of misunderstanding and disagreement. When you orient to each other with openness and vulnerability, these challenges can be a bridge to increased trust and mutuality. If not, disappointment, hurt, and emotional distance will grow.

Following is a list of what is involved when you show willingness to be vulnerable. How do these characteristics describe you?

- ❏ A spirit of openness to your partner and your situation
- ❏ Curiosity about your partner's experience
- ❏ Self-honesty about your own sensitivities
- ❏ Willingness to make and admit mistakes
- ❏ Safety and/or willingness to express your relational needs, feelings, and thoughts
- ❏ Willingness to initiate repair of your relationship

Which aspects of vulnerability are you most able to express? When?

_____

_____

_____

Which aspects of expressing vulnerability are hard for you? When?

_____

_____

_____

DOI: 10.4324/9781003476528-6

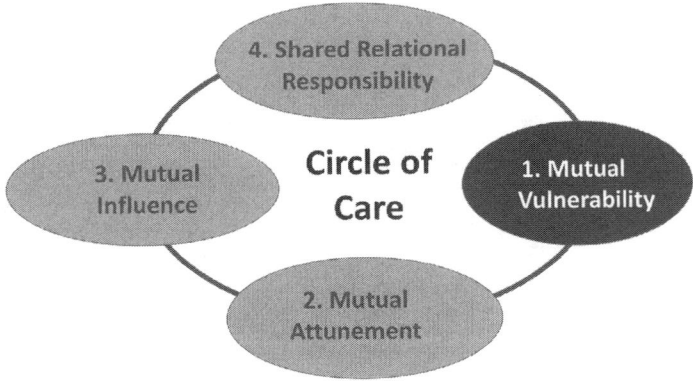

Figure 6.1 Mutual Vulnerability—First Element in the Circle of Care.

Sources of Vulnerability

Everyone experiences vulnerabilities; what they are and how you express them depends on your position in the relational flow of power, your cultural socialization, and your personal history.

> Vulnerabilities are sensitivities that arise because of your unique place in the world and your experience in family and other relationships. Like a dentist checking for soft spots or cracks in your enamel, your relational vulnerabilities are places where you are at risk of emotional pain. Your vulnerabilities are connected to the messages you have learned about how you are "supposed" to be, what you can expect from others, and your human need to be connected to and loved by others.

The emotional pain that arises when your needs to feel loved, valued, and respected are at risk is a major source of vulnerability. Following is a list of relational needs that are part of being human and some of the vulnerable feelings you may experience when they are not met or are threatened. Everyone feels these sensitivities sometimes. *Circle at least three that come up for you.*

Your vulnerabilities are also related to your felt identities (see Chapter 3) and your perceptions of what is expected of you. If you are in a position of power or have taken in social messages that you *should* be powerful, anything that could challenge your position is a potential vulnerability—for example, admitting mistakes or letting others see that you need them or are uncertain. If you are in a less powerful position, your vulnerabilities are related to the judgments and actions of those with power over you and your ability to intuit what they want—you may feel unappreciated, fearful, inadequate, or guilty for letting them down.

Relational Need	Vulnerable Feelings/Sensitivities
To be known	Feeling small, misunderstood, lost, not belonging, isolated
To be respected	Feeling humiliated, ashamed, worthless, inadequate
To be cared about	Feeling lonely, helpless, dismissed, undeserving, needy
To be validated	Feeling confused, uncertain, inadequate, incompetent, useless, a failure
To be loved	Feeling rejected, unwanted, unimportant, not good enough
To be safe	Feeling scared, hurt, worried, sad, threatened
To feel supported	Feeling overwhelmed, alone, insignificant, ineffectual

Think of a time when your need to feel loved, valued, and respected was at risk or not met.

How did your body respond? Where did you feel it?

_____

_____

_____

What did this feeling/experience say about you?

_____

_____

_____

What was your fear/sensitivity?

_____

_____

_____

What did you do?

_____

_____

_____

Think of a time when your ability to do/be what was expected of you based on your identity was at risk or compromised (for example your identity as a good mother, husband, son, employee, friend, etc.).

How did your body respond? Where did you feel it?

_____

_____

_____

What did this feeling/experience say about you?

_____

_____

_____

What was your fear/sensitivity?

_____

_____

_____

What did you do?

_____

_____

_____

Think of a time when someone hurt or threatened you or had the potential to do so.

How did your body respond? Where did you feel it?

_____

_____

_____

What did this feeling/experience say about you?

_____

_____

_____

What was your fear/sensitivity?

_____

_____

_____

What did you do?

_____

_____

_____

How Vulnerability is Expressed

Everyone experiences vulnerability, but we show it in different ways. Our research found five ways that partners express vulnerability (Knudson-Martin et al., 2021). Which way is most like you?

1 Socialized to Be Vulnerable

Katie is an example of someone society says *should* be vulnerable. These people usually identify as female or are in a socially lower power position. Like many women, Katie readily shows her vulnerability by sharing her feelings, owning her part of relationship troubles, and trying to be open to others. For example, after an argument with her partner Dan, Katie seeks to repair their connection by taking responsibility for her part and showing interest in Dan's perspective:

KATIE: (to Dan) I reacted more strongly than I should have. I was worried about my work and focused on me. I was already feeling inadequate, so when you wanted me to get ready more quickly, I lost it. I know you wanted to get there on time.

Katie's vulnerability is related to cultural messages that as a woman she is supposed to be able to maintain relationships and should not be "self-centered." Her way of expressing vulnerability reflects this stereotypic gender role. Her sensitivities include feelings such as hurt, loneliness, unworthiness, and despair when others do not reciprocate and connections fail. If this imbalance continues over time, she carries an unfair vulnerability load and may eventually try to engage her partner(s) through demands or anger, or emotionally distance herself.

2 Socialized to Appear Invulnerable

Katie's partner Dan is an example of someone society says should remain unaware of their vulnerabilities and/or hide them from others. These people usually identify as male or are in socially higher power positions. Like many men, Dan learned to distance from vulnerable feelings and project anger and strength instead. In the example with Katie, Dan did not show interest in Katie's experience. He responded to her attempt at repair by avoiding appearing weak or vulnerable himself and keeping the "blame" on her:

DAN: (to Katie) You know it's important for me to be there on time. You should plan better.

Dan's vulnerability is related to feelings that he is failing old cultural messages that as a man he should be in control and on top of things. When this happens, his chest starts to tighten and he raises his voice, but he avoids noticing what he is experiencing and is not open to Katie's perspective. His appearance of invulnerability maintains stereotypic gender roles and cuts off conversation. He may use demands, anger, distain, or distance to mask his vulnerabilities. He may worry about not being good enough or incompetent.

3 Reactive (In)vulnerability

Daryl and Hannah are examples of people for whom past experiences of trauma such as abuse or war and/or whose histories of discrimination and societal marginalization make it feel unsafe to express vulnerability. Like Katie and Dan, they receive societal messages related to their gender and social identities, but their reactions to vulnerabilities are more complex.

Hannah (who uses "they/them" pronouns) was disabled at birth and needs a wheel chair. They were sexually abused as a child and experience ongoing vulnerabilities related to their identities. When Hannah feels at risk around their needs for love, respect, and support from Daryl, they verbally attack him ferociously. Hannah is learning that this is how they try to protect themselves from additional hurt.

Daryl, who was abused by his father, responds to his relational vulnerabilities and feelings of worthlessness by emotionally shutting down. He does not want to repeat the form of masculinity modeled by his father, yet inside he sometimes feels like a failure for not being able to satisfy or control Hannah. There are many ways people who have experienced powerlessness express reactive (in)vulnerability; but like Daryl and Hannah, all react in ways that hide their emotional wounds and make them appear invulnerable but limit closeness. They may long for connection while also fearing being hurt.

4 Reactive Vulnerability

Naomi is an example of someone who responds to vulnerability and potential loss of relationship by reactively taking on all the blame in an attempt to preserve the relationship. This is a learned response to past trauma/powerlessness that exceeds "usual" female gender socialization. For example, when Naomi's partner Bente comes home from work she gives Bente a big hug and says she is glad to see her. Bente, who is feeling stressed, abruptly pushes away from Naomi. In reaction, Naomi tries to soothe Bente and expresses guilt and blame for expecting too much:

NAOMI: (*reaching out to massage Bente's shoulders*): You work so hard—you deserve to relax and not have to deal with me.
BENTE: Can't you see I'm tired!
NAOMI: I'm sorry. I can be so demanding, so insensitive—such a bad wife.

Naomi's fears around lack of worth and loss of connection are expressed in reactive vulnerability. This form of vulnerable expression puts the burden of vulnerability on Naomi while diminishing the legitimacy of her relational needs. Like all ways of expressing vulnerability, it is best understood as part of an ongoing relationship pattern that reflects each of their interpersonal histories and experiences with societal power processes.

5 Shared Vulnerability

This is when each partner can genuinely bring their sensitivities and concerns into the relationship and be interested in and open to the other without defensiveness. Shared vulnerability is an attitude, not just a skill. With awareness and practice, Naomi and Bente are learning to express shared vulnerability. Now, when Bente comes home from work similarly stressed, Naomi still gives her a big hug, but each partner responds with trust that the other is open and receptive.

BENTE: (*returns the hug*) I'm glad to see you too. I'm really feeling frazzled. I had to deal with [difficult colleague] again today and that always makes me doubt myself. I really need a bit of downtime.
NAOMI: I'm sorry you had such a hard day. Would you like to talk about it?
BENTE: Not at the moment. I need to decompress a little (smiles) and then I'd love one of your shoulder rubs—and want to hear about *your* day.

When Bente offers reciprocal vulnerability by sharing a little of her current sensitivity and shows interest in Naomi, it is easier for Naomi to feel safe in their relationship and give Bente some space. They are learning that a spirit of shared vulnerability includes curiosity and respect for the other.
Which of the five ways of expressing vulnerability is most like you?

❑ I have been socialized to maintain relationships and be the vulnerable one
❑ I have been socialized to appear invulnerable and not show weakness

❏   I protect myself from additional hurt, trauma, or discrimination by appearing invulnerable even
     though I feel unworthy or afraid inside
❏   I protect myself from additional hurt, trauma, or discrimination by carrying all the vulnerability,
     responsibility, and blame in my relationship(s)
❏   My partner(s) and I usually share vulnerability and efforts to maintain connection

> **List some examples of how you generally express vulnerability (or maintain the appearance of invulnerability)**
>
> _____
>
> _____
>
> _____
>
> _____
>
> _____

Even if socialization and/or experiences of trauma, abuse, or discrimination have made it difficult
for you and your partner(s) to regularly share vulnerability, there are almost certainly times when
you have experienced it.

> **Think of a time when you and your partner(s) shared vulnerability. What did you do? What did
> your partner do? How did it affect you?**
>
> _____
>
> _____
>
> _____
>
> _____
>
> _____

Turn Toward

Sometimes fear of being hurt or weak may cause you to build walls, to detach, to appear invulnerable, or react with defensiveness or shame. Or perhaps you just go along to keep things smooth,
hiding much of who you are and what you feel to keep the peace or avoid rejection. To relate
instead with a spirit of openness and vulnerability, you need to remember only one thing: *turn
toward*.

Turn Toward Your Relational Needs

Turning toward means acknowledging that you and your partner are relational beings who choose
to be in relationship. When you turn toward your partner, as Bente did when she hugged back, you
are saying "our relationship matters—you matter."

Now and in the next few days, be aware of your relational needs:

To be known _____

To be respected _____

To be cared about _____

To be validated _____

To be loved _____

To be safe _____

To be supported _____

If you tend to keep the appearance of invulnerability, on the list above note a way you could share your vulnerability around each of these sensitivities with your partner (a worry, fear, weaknesses, uncertainty, etc.). For example, Bente let Naomi know that she doubted herself in the interaction with her colleague.

If you tend to openly express vulnerability (your love, your worries, your faults, etc.), this is a good step toward connection. On the list above, note a way you turn toward each of these needs with your partner. For example, Katie let Dan know that she was feeling inadequate and admitted that she reacted more strongly than she should have.

Turn Toward Your Partner(s)

Develop the habit of saying or doing something that initiates connection. It can be as simple as looking toward your partner when they are talking or literally reaching out to them. This is easy when you feel safe, valued, and loved. But even in the best of relationships, there are moments when your first impulse may be to pull away or take a defensive stance. I remember when my husband and I were arguing while we were building a house. He turned to me and said, "I love you; we'll get through this." That reminder of our connection changed everything.

Examples of turning toward include:

- Responding to differences or anger with curiosity about your partner's perspective
- Sharing what you are feeling or worried about
- Admitting mistakes
- Asking for your partner's advice or input
- Expressing your love and caring
- Physical affection (without demands or expectations)
- Showing interest in your partner's life

If your relationship is going through a hard time, or the old rules for marriage have invaded your life, *turning toward* can sometimes seem like a risk. The good news for Katie and Dan is that Katie has not given up on bringing a spirit of vulnerability to the relationship. Instead, she turns toward Dan by telling him how important he is to her and shares some of her sensitive feelings (rather than attack or demand). She uses words that convey her personal experience, which helps to engage Dan in what matters to her:

KATIE: I can't get what happened last night out of my mind. I feel anxious and worried. You are so important to me. I don't know what I'd do if we drifted apart.

DAN: What do you mean drifted apart? I think you're making a mountain out of a molehill.

KATIE: (*sticking to her personal experience rather than defending herself*) I feel disconnected from you sometimes. Last night I was freaked out about work. Thinking about you being there for me made me feel better. But you were so worked up about getting going, that I shut down.

DAN: I didn't know—I want you to talk to me; to be there for you.

Katie asks Dan to do this workbook with her as a way to move forward together. Though Dan resists at first, the genuineness of Katie's vulnerability and his own desire for a better relationship moves him.

If you tend to take an invulnerable position, the turning point is on you. You need to take a lead in turning toward each other. Katie's vulnerability was important, but the relationship could not move toward mutual care until Dan took steps to initiate connection. Even small moves toward connection, such as showing interest in your partner's viewpoints can make a huge difference.

If you tend to show your vulnerability, but your partner doesn't, the best thing you can do is to behave how you prefer to be in your relationship. Use the Circle of Care as your guide. Oftentimes, as in the example of Katie and Dan, when you maintain a spirit of openness and share what is actually happening for you, your partner will respond by also turning toward you. If over time your partner maintains the appearance of invulnerability and is not able to reciprocally turn toward you, you may need to let your partner know where you stand regarding the imbalance—another vulnerable step that should still focus on your personal experience rather than attack. This honesty, perhaps with the help of a therapist or counselor, can provide an impetus for change. What kind of change depends on how your partner responds.

If you both tend to take an invulnerable position, either of you can initiate a turn toward your partner. A mutually supportive, loving relationship is one of best ways to heal from prior abuse and hurt. In the case of Daryl and Hannah, Daryl decides that the next time Hannah explodes in anger, he will realize that Hannah's anger is a mask for their vulnerability. He will turn toward Hannah rather than distance from them. He will use Hannah's anger as an opening to be with them and explore their differences. Daryl begins by admitting to himself that his withdrawal in the face of anger is not helpful and probably hurts Hannah. When Hannah attacks him for "not caring," Daryl moves toward them:

DARYL: (*feeling the pull to shut down, but staying present*): Help me understand, Hannah. I love you. It hurts my heart to see you so unhappy.

HANNAH: (*interested but mistrustful*) Well! Your heart must hurt a lot then.

DARYL: (*persisting in staying present*) It does. Yours must too. Help me understand what you need from me.

HANNAH: (*after a pause*) I think I need to trust that you're not going away.

Daryl's turn toward Hannah opens conversation about their prior hurts and how they learned to protect themselves. They make a pact to help each other react differently and to be there for each other. With a number of ups and downs and the Circle of Care as a guide, their increasingly shared vulnerability helps them build trust—trust that when problems happen, they can get through them together.

Make a Plan

What is something you can do to turn toward your partner?

_____

_____

_____

When is this likely to happen? Describe the situation.

_____

_____

_____

When you think about initiating your plan to turn toward your partner, what is your fear or vulnerability?

_____

_____

_____

What will you need to do to stay with your plan to turn toward? What will help you stay *with* your partner, rather than resorting to anger, demands, or distance?

_____

_____

_____

_____

Possible Bumps Along the Way

The understanding of yourself and your partner that you gain as you go through the activities in this book will make it easier to open your hearts to each other—to build trust by turning toward each other with shared vulnerability. As is always true in learning something new, there are sometimes bumps along the way. Following are some that could come up. You can get through them when you each persist in *turning toward*.

Your Bodily Responses to Risk and Harm

Our bodies are designed to turn toward each other in the face of stress or danger. But if others have let you down or hurt you in the past—whether by people close to you or through injustice at the societal level—your body may have learned to avoid pain by shutting down or defending against closeness. These responses tend to kick in even when they are no longer necessary. You need to recognize these internal messages and intentionally override them. The emotional map provided in Appendix E may be helpful.

Anger

Anger is an important message about your situation. *If anger is your usual form of response* to vulnerability, you need to look under the anger for the softer relational needs and sensitives that anger is hiding. In other words, anger is an early-warning system that tells you to look for the real issue. When anger bubbles up, that is your clue to pause and look at what anger is saying about what you fear and need.

If your partner tended to hide (or not feel) anger in the past, this may be because she did not previously feel safe enough or entitled to express anger. When you soften and take steps toward each other, it is possible that her anger will now pop out. If this happens, do not withdraw or respond with anger. She needs to know you are interested in her and willing to be vulnerable enough to hear it. It may be hard to stay present and take in what she says through anger, but when you do, you open new pathways for connection.

Persistence of Gender Patterns

Even when you do not believe male interests are more important than female ones, this old relational idea can easily persist in your responses to each other. For example, when men express some of their vulnerabilities, their needs and interests can take up all the relational space without either of you realizing it. If you are socialized as male, you may unconsciously expect it. If you are socialized as female, you may feel grateful for what he has shared and automatically focus on him, letting go of some or most of your needs and interests. Keep the idea of reciprocity and mutual vulnerability as a guide. If you are a man or otherwise in a more powerful position, extra awareness and intentionally turning toward your partner's interests will help.

Power Struggles

Power struggles are a sign each of you is safeguarding something important to you. Most likely you are each avoiding hurt or protecting your identity. It may also be a sign that one or each of you is resisting the old gender pattern that women accommodate men. Power struggles also indicate that you each care what your partner thinks and about what happens between you. Like Daryl in the earlier example, either of you can break the impasse with curiosity about your partner's perspective/input or by sharing what you are worried about, admitting your part in your struggles, and/or expressing your love and affection.

Oftentimes, the struggle is about who will be vulnerable first. This is understandable, since neither of you feels fully safe. Regardless of who starts, each of you must turn toward the other in order to build trust based on mutual vulnerability. Gender and other societal power differences make it likely that one of you is holding on to a power position, while the other is resisting a one-down position and pushing to be heard (see Chapter 5). If you are [intentionally or not] in a more powerful position, your shift to vulnerability will be an essential step toward the mutually loving relationship you want.

Hurt and Accountability

Letting yourself be aware of how you have hurt someone you love or the ways you have contributed to disappointment in the relationship involves opening yourself to vulnerabilities. The temptation, especially if you are not used to being in a vulnerable position, is to want your partner to move from their hurt quickly once you've acknowledged it. But it may take time. You may need to sit with vulnerability while your partner begins to trust that it is safe to be open and connected to you. It is worth it.

Stepping Toward Mutual Vulnerability

Doing the activities and conversations in this book means you have already been taking steps toward mutual vulnerability. You have shown openness to learning about your sensitivities and curiosity about your partner's experience. You are willing to try something new.

Pause for a moment to consider what this says about you.

What is it about you that makes you open to being vulnerable?

_____

_____

_____

Who would not be surprised to learn that you are open to being vulnerable? Why?

_____

_____

_____

Conversation 6

This conversation will help you deepen your commitment to mutual vulnerability. Like all the conversations in this book, it is structured to create safety and mutuality. You can express vulnerability without being attacked or criticized, and there is space for each of you. As you begin, orient to your conversational partner(s) with curiosity and openness to learning.

Orient with curiosity

- Make yourself comfortable and close your eyes
- Be aware of your breath as it gently goes in and out
- Be aware of any tension, worry, or judgment. Gently let them go
- Open your eyes. Be aware of your conversational partner(s)
- Be aware of the larger world connected to each of you
- Be aware of any tension, worry, or judgment. Gently let them go
- Be aware of your interest in knowing your partner(s)

This activity follows the same conversational structure used in the previous chapters. Each of you responds to the first question for up to two minutes; then you move on to the second and so on. Listeners do not interrupt or comment. When speaking, take time to let your thoughts evolve. Alternate who begins the next question. If you are doing the exercise without a partner, write your answers and then read them aloud to yourself. It is important to hear your voice.

1 Share a story about what you learned growing up about the expression of vulnerability? What societal and relational messages were involved? What is important about it to you today?

2 Share a story about a time when your needs to be respected or validated were at risk or not met, but the situation did not involve your partner. How did you respond? How has this experience, or experiences like it, affected you?

3   Share a story about a time when your needs to be loved, cared about, and safe were at risk or not met, but did not involve your partner. How did your respond? How has this experience, or experiences like it, affected you?

4   Share a story about a time your partner made you feel loved, cared about, respected, or validated. What did your partner do that was especially meaningful to you? How has this experience affected you?

5   Share a story about a relational sensitivity that you recently experienced with your partner. What was your worry or fear? What was your hope?

6   What has moved you as you listened to your conversational partner's stories today? What new awareness or questions are coming up for you? (Partner does not answer.)

7   Share a plan to "turn toward" mutual vulnerability that you commit to initiating. What will be challenging for you? Why is this step important?

Additional Resources

Build your capacity for vulnerability. You can copy the worksheet in Appendix I at the back of the book or download it by visiting www.routledge.com/9781032759890 and clicking on the link that says "Support Material." Use it to create a plan to enhance your capacity for mutual vulnerability. For each example of "turning toward" your partner, describe at least one new vulnerable action you will take. Do at least two each week. In the third column, describe what you learned from taking this action. Print additional copies to track your capacity over time.

Vulnerability and the Man Box. Appendix J (at the back of the book or at www.routledge.com/9781032759890) includes a quote from Mark Greene's (2018) *The Little #MeToo Book for Men.* Use it as a stimulus to reflect on "the man box" and mutual vulnerability in your life. The book "exposes the brutal price that man box culture extracts from men and women worldwide... and invites men to step out of silence and isolation and into a better future" (back cover). It is short, inexpensive, and easy to read. I highly recommend it.

Chapter 7

Attune to One Another

Attuned communication is a major reason healthy relationships are so good for you (and bad relationships are not). When mutual, each of you feels felt, known. It is the opposite of feeling isolated, alone, and unimportant. Mutual attunement, which builds on mutual vulnerability (Chapter 6), is the second element of the Circle of Care (see Figure 7.1). In this chapter, you will learn what is involved in mutual attunement and take four simple steps to practice it.

What is Attunement, and Why is It Important?

When you attune to your partner, you proactively notice what your partner feels and needs rather than passively waiting to be told. Mutual attunement is literally your mind/body linking with another's. *Mirror neurons*, nerve cells inside *your* body, take in and reflect what is going on for your partner (Figure 7.2). Your mirror neurons imitate what they are experiencing such that *you* feel it inside. Another word for this is *being with*.

When you and your partner are mutually attuned, you may not necessarily agree, but you "get" each other—you feel felt. This is a calming experience that allows you to feel connected and safe, that you belong. Interpersonal neurobiologists, such as Daniel Siegel (2020) in *The Developing Mind: How Relationships and the Brain Interact to Shape Who We Are*, teach that we need this interconnectedness to manage our emotions, flexibly adapt to change, and thrive.

> When you were upset or stimulated as a child, you needed an attuned response from your caregivers to help you manage your emotions. This helped you find the sweet spot between overreacting (chaos) and underreacting (rigidity). As adults, responsive mutually attuned connection remains a necessary touchstone and source of support.

How do you know if attunement is mutual?

- ❏ Each of you pauses to notice the other
- ❏ You each feel "with" your partner
- ❏ You each thoughtfully respond to your partner's felt experience
- ❏ Each of you feels comforted, less stressed

The following examples will help you explore how mutual attunement works in your relationship.

Example 1: Mutual Attunement

It is 4:00 pm. Alejandro walks in the door after a long day delivering produce to restaurants. He has been on a tight supply schedule since 7:00 am and feels beat. Joanie has been home all day with their teething infant and a toddler who has just learned the delight of saying "no!" Joanie is exhausted.

DOI: 10.4324/9781003476528-7

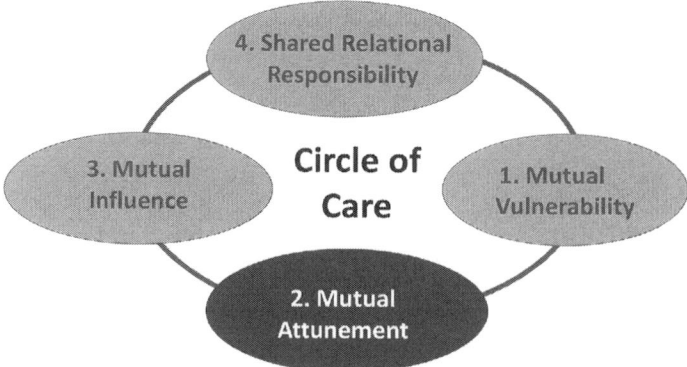

Figure 7.1 Mutual Attunement—Second Element in the Circle of Care

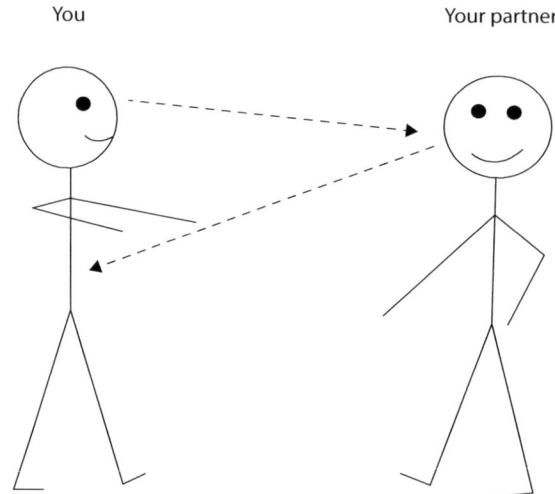

Figure 7.2 Attunement—Process of "Being With"

Alejandro gives Joanie a quick kiss, then looks directly at her. He remembers that the baby is teething and shares a compassionate smile:

ALEJANDRO: How's it been going? Has Miko had a hard day?
JOANIE: (looks at Alejandro and smiles wryly): We had a lot of fussing today. And every time I picked up Miko, Maya wanted my attention.

Alejandro notices the tiredness in Joanie's eyes and envisions Miko crying while Maya is pulling at her for attention. He begins to feel the tug inside that Joanie must have been experiencing—the love for their children while also just wanting some peace.

ALEJANDRO: Oh, honey (*compassionate pause*) I know how much you love these little guys, and still, you could have used a little peace.
JOANIE: (*feels felt and begins to relax a little*) You got that right. I do love them so much, but sometimes....

*Joanie looks at Alejandro. As she thinks about **his** day, she can feel the pressure on him to make all the deliveries on time.*

JOANIE: And what about you? It was raining pretty hard today; that must have made it difficult to keep on schedule.

ALEJANDRO: (*feels felt, and the tension in his back begins to recede*) Yeah. It was tight. Traffic was hell. (*Looks at her, feels connected, and reaches for the baby.*) I'm glad to be home. Here, let me sit with Miko for a bit. (*Turns to their daughter*). Maya, can you "read" Daddy and Miko a story?

The time before dinner can be challenging, especially if you have young children. What did you notice about how Alejandro and Joanie attuned to each other in this busy moment?

_____

_____

_____

What do you think made their connection possible?

_____

_____

_____

In an intimate relationship, there is often a rapid exchange of information as each of you pick up on what the other is experiencing and adjust. In this exchange, Joannie and Alejandro did not spend a lot of time in in-depth conversation, as they sometimes might. But in their brief encounter, *each was changed by the other.* They began to relax, to feel less alone. Their energy began to flow in more positive directions.

Alejandro and Joannie did four things to attune:

1 They focused on each other.
2 They were emotionally open and aware.
3 They practiced empathic imagination.
4 They thoughtfully responded.

Notice how the couple in the next example does not employ these attuned practices.

Example 2: Lack of Attunement

It is 5:30 pm. Albert walks in the door, kicks off his shoes, drops into the recliner, and settles in to watch the news. He is exhausted after teaching science all day and coaching the 6th grade basketball team after school. A few minutes later, Camille comes in with their kids, Suzie in first grade and Tyrone in third. Camille has picked them up from their after-school day care. While she empties their backpacks, she thinks about the report she still needs to finish for the sales meeting tomorrow. She sighs, pops a frozen pizza into the oven and begins to prepare a salad. Albert yells a "hello" from the family room:

ALBERT: Hey! How're you doing? Need help?
CAMILLE: (*sighs*) I got it. It's just pizza and salad. Tyrone has a spelling test tomorrow. Can you help him go over the words after dinner?
ALBERT: Sure. No problem. (*Turns back to the television.*)

After dinner, Camille cleans up and Albert helps the kids get ready for bed. After they are tucked in, Albert grades papers and Camille works on her report.

What did you notice about how the ways Albert and Camille interacted differ from the first couple?

_____

_____

_____

_____

Both couples have long days and young children. Both are coordinating with each other in raising the children. But Albert and Camile have fallen out of the habit of tuning in:

1   They did not pause to focus on each other.
2   They were not emotionally open and present with each other.
3   They did not use their mirror neurons to take in/imagine the other.
4   They responded to each other by rote or habit.

Camille and Albert are at risk of drifting apart and each feels increasingly worn out.

Are you more like the first couple or the second couple? How?

_____

_____

_____

_____

_____

What Limits Mutual Attunement?

Like vulnerability, mutual attunement is as much an attitude as a skill. Societal messages that emphasize individuality, competition, dominance, and being right get in the way of focusing on others. Partners like

Alejandro and Joanie (Example 1) do not need to actively focus on each other all the time; that would be impossible. But they have each developed an "orientation to other" that counteracts the culture of individualism (see Appendix G). Alejandro did not have to tell himself to pause to focus on Joanie and the children even though he was tired. He had developed an attuned orientation that made focusing on them, and the benefits he received back, second nature.

In contrast, Albert and Camille are so focused on surviving in the outside world, they do not stop to focus on each other. As a Black couple they learned to pull together to deal with the extra stress and marginalization they face in society (see Cowdery et al, 2009). Camille is aware of the extra scrutiny Black men experience and tends to excuse Albert at home. Both adhere to the myth of the strong Black woman, and overlook Camille's needs for comfort and support.

> An imbalance in attunement is common. If power tends to flow to you (see chapter 5), developing an attuned mindset may require your conscious intention. Societal based power differences built into old gender rules and disparities based on income, social status, race, ethnicity, sexuality, abilities, and other factors affect who tends to focus on whom. Madelyn and Byron (below) are an example.

Example 3: Unbalanced Attunement

Madelyn and Byron, a White couple in their early 60s with grown children from prior relationships, met in seminary where each was making a mid-life career change. They have similar jobs as ministers, and were attracted to their shared commitment to helping others and making the world a better place. They have lots of conversations about their work and what is happening in their communities and society. Yet they bring very different power positions into their relationship, which limits mutual attunement. Byron was raised in an affluent family and was socialized to be a "go-getter, on top of the world." Though he changed careers to live more consistently with his humanitarian values, as a former male CFO (chief financial officer) he is used to being in charge and respected. Madelyn was raised in a working-class family. She has been working outside the home since her father died when she was 15 and has frequently faced harassment or marginalization due to her gender. She readily attunes to others and expects/hopes that Byron will also attune to her. Last night is typical:

It is nearly 9:00 pm. Madelyn has just come home from a contentious meeting with the Church Council. Byron is reading in the living room.

BYRON : (*looks up*): Hi. How'd it go?

MADELYN: (*sits in the chair next to him*) Not good. (sighs and describes a conflict between the council members) It was all I could do to stay respectful and keep them focused.

Madelyn is feeling stressed and could use an understanding ear.

BYRON: Church councils are like that. (*He suggests how he would handle it.*)

MADELYN: (*feels even more tired*). Yeah. Thanks. I appreciate your perspective, but I think my situation is a little different (*Attempts to share what she is feeling*). I feel so dismissed by [two of the council members].

BYRON: It'll be better in the morning. (*Turns on the television.*)

MADELYN: (feels dismissed by Byron). Yeah. Maybe.

They watch their usual night time program, then prepare for bed.

BYRON: (to Madelyn, who is already in bed) I'm going to take a shower and then go downstairs to read a little more.

MADELYN: OK. Goodnight. Would you turn off the bedroom light when you're finished?

BYRON: OK. (*A little later he leaves without turning out the light.*)

Madelyn needs to feel felt, that Byron understands (or at least is trying to understand) what was stressful for her. Instead of attuning to what it is like for Madelyn in her setting, Byron responds with advice based on his experience, then later "forgets" to do what she asked. By themselves these are small things, but they are part of an ongoing imbalance in the relationship that often leaves Madelyn without the benefit of attuned support.

Though Madelyn is beginning to feel a little disillusioned with their relationship, she is still generally attuned to Byron. For example, the next morning Byron has just finished a phone call with his son, Denny.

MADELYN: (*notices tension in Byron's jaw*) How was the conversation with Denny?

BYRON: OK. Denny is working so many hours at the practice; he's hardly ever home.

MADELYN: (*sensing the concern in his voice*) You're worried about him...

BYRON: Yeah. (*starts to relax a bit*) I know I have to let him live his own life, but I worry he's making the same mistakes I made.

MADELYN: (*beginning to feel his worry*) You love him. You want him to be happy (puts her arm around him)—and you feel responsible?

Byron sighs and settles into the hug. He talks for a few minutes about what he wishes he had done differently as a father, then begins to gather his things for work.

BYRON: (feels better) Thanks. I love you. I'll be home early today.

When Madelyn focuses on Byron with the desire to "get" what he is experiencing, her mirror neurons help her feel Byron's worry and remorse. She is able to be *with* Byron. Though it is only for a few moments, Byron feels the impact—is positively changed by Madelyn—as he starts his day.

Are you more likely to respond to your partner similarly to Byron or more like Madelyn?

_____

_____

_____

As you consider how you attune to your partner, what thoughts come to mind?

_____

_____

_____

As you consider how your partner attunes to you, what thoughts come to mind?

_____

_____

_____

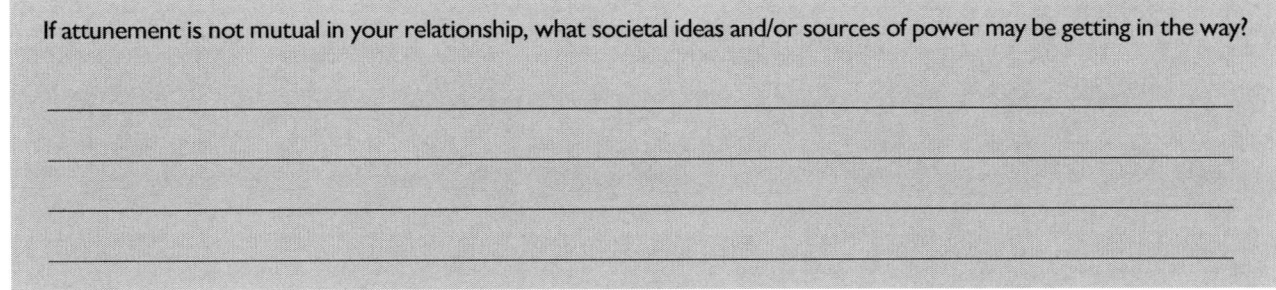

If attunement is not mutual in your relationship, what societal ideas and/or sources of power may be getting in the way?

_____

_____

_____

_____

Sometimes attunement is so out of balance, that one partner carries all the effort to maintain the relationship, often at an expense to their own well-being. Note the imbalance between Esther and Wilma in their interview with Naveen Jonathan (2009, p. 94) about their relationship:

ESTHER: It almost makes me feel like our relationship does not exist. I would be willing to be more out, but Wilma is not ready for that.

WILMA: I'm comfortable the way things are. Why do we have to come out, just because it suits you?

ESTHER: It's not that I want to force us to come out, but I really feel that it would give our relationship more value … if others knew.

WILMA: Esther has the choice to be with me. If she's not happy, I would rather she find someone else.

Wilma shows no interest in Esther's perspective. Though her unattuned response is connected to unfairness in the larger society, she seems unlikely to take steps to develop mutual attunement that would enable them to address the discrimination together.

More often, when partners such as Byron become aware that they are not as attuned to their partners as they wish—or each partner realizes they are no longer as focused on the other as they used to be—learning to practice attunement is not as hard as you might think.

Steps to Mutual Attunement

Attunement is not magic. As shown in Figure 7.3, four elements are involved: (1) intentionally focus on the other; (2) open yourself to be emotionally present; (3) practice empathic imagination; and (4) thoughtfully respond. Your goal is to feel what your partner feels, to be on the same wavelength. To get started, take each step one at a time. After a while, these steps will become more automatic.

I Intentionally Focus on Your Partner

You create the neural pathways in your brain/body by what you focus on. Attuning to your partner begins with a decision to focus on them. It is an intentional act. If you have not been in the habit of focusing on your partner, you do not have a neural path readily connecting you. But the more you focus on your partner, the more the neural connection will grow. Like a path through the forest or a meadow, the first time through is charting new territory, but once you've walked it a few times it is easier to follow. After a while, you only need to point yourself in the right direction to move toward attunement.

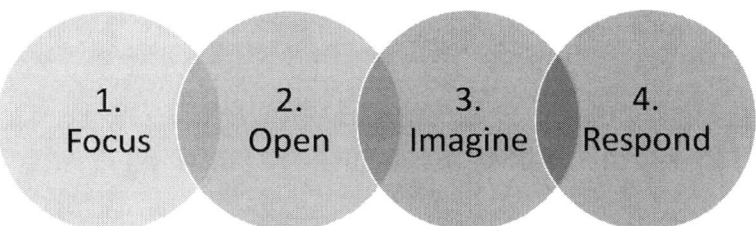

Figure 7.3 Elements of Attunement.

Exercise 1: Focus

Pause right now. Whether your partner is in the room with you or somewhere across the world, focus your attention on your partner. Picture your partner. Where are they? What are they doing? What signals are present in the way their body moves, their facial expressions? Picture the details.

Describe the scene so that someone else could see it:

_____

_____

_____

_____

_____

_____

_____

What did you have to do to move your focus to your partner?

_____

_____

_____

As you focused on your partner, what did you notice about yourself?

_____

_____

_____

If you are not in the habit of attuning to your partner as much as you'd like, intentionally take regular time to focus on them, to notice the details. Answer the same questions as above. As in developing any skill, repetition is important.

2 Open Yourself to Be Emotionally Present

Be receptive to what is happening. Be careful of preconceived ideas and judgements. When these come up for you, gently push them away. Focus on being *with* your partner. Let yourself be curious about what is happening for them. For example, Byron is practicing being focused on and open to Madelyn. The next time she starts to tell him about her frustration with members of the Church Council, he is aware that he thinks she is not assertive enough. He feels the pull to give advice, but gently pushes these thoughts aside and focuses on her. As she speaks, he notices the tension on her face and that her voice is getting higher pitched. He finds himself interested in what is happening for her and focuses on what she is focused on. He says, "trying to get [two Church Council members] to settle down is really hard, stressful." This encourages Madelyn to say more, with more detail. They are now focusing on the same thing, which is supportive and carries the potential for healing.

It is harder if your partner is distressed or upset about something regarding you. This is a vulnerable position. You want to *be with* your partner, but have to be open to the possibility that you've hurt the person you love. You may feel misunderstood or the need to defend yourself. If you do not first take in what your partner is experiencing, you'll not be able to resolve the disagreement. For example, when Madelyn says to Byron, "I know this seems like a small thing, but I felt hurt when you didn't remember to shut off the light last night," Byron has to gently push aside his irritation at himself for forgetting and his sense that she is building this way out of proportion. He worries that she thinks he is a bad person. He turns to Madelyn, apologizes, and says, "I can see this is important to you." She tells him more.

Exercise 2: Open

Notice a time when you partner is sending signals that seem especially meaningful. It could be something positive or something distressing or even something routine. Let yourself be open to your partner.

What did you need to do to be open? What preconceived thoughts or personal reactions did you need to get out of the way?

_____

_____

_____

_____

How did you know that you and your partner were focusing on the same thing?

_____

_____

_____

_____

If you find this exercise challenging or know that you are not in the habit of opening to your partner, repeat the exercise multiple times. Get familiar with what it feels like to open yourself. Take stock of the challenges that might be getting in your way.

3 Practice Empathic Imagination

Now that you and your partner are focusing on the same thing, you can more actively engage. Your mirror neurons will help you feel what your partner feels. But to get it right, you need to draw on what you see and what you know about your partner's world to ask yourself what is happening—to *imagine* what it is like to be your partner at this moment. Empathy arises in the process of seeking to "get" your partner and will guide what you are curious about. The usefulness of your mirror neurons depends of three things:

- Your genuine interest in and curiosity about your partner
- Your ability to tune into yourself to access what your mirror neurons are telling you
- Your ability to distinguish your experience from your partner's

Byron has developed his capacity to use his mirror neurons in other settings. When he was a CFO, he was good at determining the interests of various partners when making a deal. As a clergyman, he is good at tuning into members of his congregation. When he first met Madelyn, he could empathically imagine her world as they focused together on their dreams of service. But he has not developed the habit of stopping to imagine Madelyn as a person now. He tends to think of her experience as like his own.

As Madelyn talks about how members of the Church Council seem dismissive of her, Bryon tries to imagine what it is like to be Madelyn, to feel dismissed. He realizes that it is not a common feeling for him, and if he does feel slighted, he has ways to assert his authority. He doesn't know what it feels like to be Madelyn. "Say more about being dismissed," he says. "What is that like for you?" As Madelyn describes how the council members ignore her and talk over her, Byron begins to imagine what it is like to hold her position of authority but not always be respected in it.

Exercise 3: Imagine

Pick one of the times that you practiced being open to your partner. Imagine that you are your partner. From your partner's point of view, write a journal entry about this emotionally important experience. Write in first person, as though you are your partner. Describe what is happening, what your partner is feeling, and what it means to your partner.

_____

_____

_____

_____

_____

_____

_____

_____

What did you have to do to imagine your partner, to access your mirror neurons?

_____

_____

_____

What questions or curiosities about your partner's experience came up for you?

_____

_____

_____

How is empathically imagining your partner different than your own experience in a similar situation?

_____

_____

_____

_____

If you have not been as attuned to your partner as you would like, practice imagining what is happening for her/him/them. Intentionally focus on your partner and open yourself to their experience, then draw on your mirror neurons and what you know about their situation to imagine what it is like for your partner. *Repeat this exercise at least once a week for a month* —write a journal entry from the perspective of your partner and use the previous reflective questions to help you distinguish your experience from your partner's.

4 Thoughtfully Respond

When you allow your internal state to align with another's, you will respond to them in a genuine and compassionate manner. You will be curious about what is meaningful to them. You may *name what you hear* and respond with questions/comments that clarify or invite further reflection, such as:

- Tell me more
- Am I understanding correctly?
- What else?
- I wonder?

You stay curious and resist telling the other person what to do. You take actions that are supportive and helpful. If the issue involves you, you will be accountable for your behavior and responsive to your partner's concerns. Byron found himself wondering if Madelyn also felt dismissed when he ignored her requests, such as to shut off the light:

BYRON: (*thoughtfully*) I'm wondering if you also feel dismissed by me when I don't seem to listen or take you seriously.

MADELYN: (*feels a surge of connection*) Yes! That's it. It's really important to me that you take me seriously. It was one of the reasons I fell in love with you.

Attuned responsiveness such as this is what you and your partner each need for ongoing health and well-being. Madelyn feels better, but so does Byron. This grounding in mutual connection helps you overcome other sources of disconnection, distress, and fear.

Exercise 4: Thoughtfully Respond

The next time you practice imaginatively attuning to your partner, notice what your attunement makes you curious about or interested in. Ask you partner to tell you more.

What did you feel moved to do or say?

_____

_____

_____

_____

What enabled you to be thoughtfully responsive, rather than defensive or responding on auto-pilot?

_____

_____

_____

_____

How did your partner respond? What do you think your attuned response meant to your partner?

_____

_____

_____

_____

If you had difficulty thoughtfully responding to your partner from a place of attuned connection, use this as an opportunity to reflect on yourself. What ideas or worries about yourself and/or your partner get in the way? Keep experimenting. Learning a new way of orienting to your partner can take time.

If your partner did not react positively to your thoughtful response, remain curious. What did you miss? What do you still need to understand? Keep practicing, taking care to maintain genuine interest in your partner and to honestly reflect on what you bring to the situation.

If your partner is not also trying to attune to you, you may need the help of a couple's therapist or counselor. Mutual attunement is a two-way street.

Positive Cycle of Mutuality

Learning to practice mutual attunement creates avenues for flexibility, growth, and well-being based on care, love, and connection. Each person benefits not only from being attuned to, but also through the process of connecting to another.

Conversation 7

This conversation will help you explore mutual attunement. Like all the conversations in this book, it is structured to facilitate a shared experience. Begin by orienting to your conversational partner(s) with curiosity and openness to learning.

Orient with curiosity

- Make yourself comfortable and close your eyes
- Be aware of your breath as it gently goes in and out
- Be aware of any tension, worry, or judgment. Gently let them go
- Open your eyes. Be aware of your conversational partner(s).
- Be aware of the larger world connected to each of you

- Be aware of any tension, worry, or judgment. Gently let them go
- Be aware of your interest in knowing your partner(s)

This activity follows the same conversational structure used in the previous chapters. Each of you responds to the first question for up to two minutes; then you move on to the second and so on. Listeners do not interrupt or comment. When speaking, take time to let your thoughts evolve. Alternate who begins the next question. If you are doing the exercise without a partner, write your answers and then read them aloud to yourself. It is important to hear your voice.

1   What do you know about yourself that says you are interested in and able to attune to others. Share a story that shows why this is true. Who else knows this about you?

2   Share an example of when you were able to successfully attune to your partner. What did you do to create attunement? How did you know?

3   Tell a story about your partner from their point of view. What is important to your partner in this story? What did you need to do to take in your partner's experience?

4   What are you learning about the next steps for you in practicing mutual attunement with your partner? Where do you get stuck? What ideas related to your identity or society get in the way? Give examples.

5   How will you and your relationship be different when you are better able to responsively attune to each other? How will you know? What will you see? What will you be doing? What will your partner be doing?

6   As you listened to your conversational partner(s) today, what new thoughts or questions have come up for you? Why are these important? (Partner does not answer.)

7   What do you want your partner to know about your commitment to mutual attunement? What does this commitment say about you? Why is this important to you?

Additional Resources

Steps Toward Mutual Attunement. Copy Appendix K from the back of the book or download it by visiting www.routledge.com/9781032759890 and clicking on the link that says "Support Material." Use it to list what you do when you successfully enact each of the four steps toward mutual attunement. It is a way to personalize the steps and document your progress. You can make multiple copies and repeat as often as you wish. Alternatively, you can use the worksheet as a place for you and your partner to document your commitment to mutual attunement in your own words.

Chapter 8

Open to Influence

Do you believe relationships should mutually benefit each partner? That good relationships involve reciprocal give and take? That they should be fair? These processes of mutual influence sound straightforward, but happen in a multitude of ways, many of which you may hardly notice or think about. Examples include:

- Which topics get discussed
- How daily schedules are organized
- The impact of your feelings and interests on your partner
- Who defines the situation, what's "real"
- How decisions are made
- How responsibilities are divided
- Who listens, notices, remembers
- Whose contributions/ideas are minimized or supported
- Automatic or taken-for-granted accommodations to the other
- How conflict is addressed
- Availability to one another

These kinds of relational back and forth are a daily part of life. Yet odds are that you stepped into your relationship without training, or even discussion, of how to mutually influence each other. Even if you're lucky and mutual influence was modeled for you, the old rules for relationships and messages from a competitive, individualistic society, easily get in the way.

In this chapter you'll learn how successful couples practice the third element of the Circle of Care, mutual influence (see Figure 8.1). You'll learn how to keep gender and other sources of power imbalances from taking over influence processes in your relationship and begin to create influence patterns grounded in mutuality.

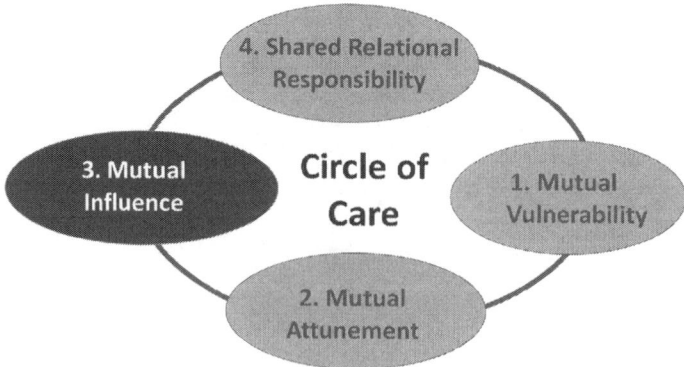

Figure 8.1 Mutual Influence—Element Three in the Circle of Care.

DOI: 10.4324/9781003476528-8

What is Mutual Influence?

Influence is the ability to have an impact on your partner and how your relationship works. When mutual, each of you can engage the other in issues that matter to you and your well-being. Each of your interests is expressed and reflected in ongoing relationship processes, such as those listed at the beginning of this chapter. Each of you accommodates and adapts to the other. You each have an impact on the other and look out for the other's well-being, as well as your own.

Pause for a moment. Think about your partner.

Quickly list at least ten things that matter to your partner.

_____

_____

_____

_____

_____

How do you know?

_____

_____

_____

How does reflecting on your partner's interests and priorities affect you? What are you curious to know more about? What are you moved to do?

_____

_____

_____

_____

_____

Mutual influence is directly related to mutual attunement. You do not just "give-in" to keep the peace; you are mutually touched by the other. You reciprocally influence what each of you feels, knows, and understands. Recall from Chapter 7 that in this attuned process, you literally feel each other and respond from this attuned sense of knowing. Even though you may not always agree, your partner is there for you, responsive to you and your well-being. This is why *openness* to influence is so important.

Why Influence Can Be Tricky

All the sources of power imbalances you learned about in this book (see Chapter 5) affect openness to being influenced. You may have learned that being influenced means you are not strong enough, not man enough; that accepting influence means you're not in charge, not in control. Or you may have learned that it is selfish to express your needs and interests, that it is your job to support others and make them feel good. And, if you've been hurt or abused by the power of others, letting yourself be open to influence can feel risky; you may have learned to protect yourself by preemptively taking control and/or emotionally distancing yourself.

Cultural messages about self-reliance, independence, and competitiveness that tell you to stand your ground, know what you want, and not let your ideas be influenced by others also get in the way of mutual influence (see Chapter 2). No wonder influence processes between you and your partner(s) can be tricky! There may be a lot going on under the surface.

> What messages about how and whether to be influenced by others have you taken in? Where did you learn them—from society? media? from friends, family, colleagues?
>
> _____
> _____
> _____
> _____
> _____

A few examples will shed light on some of the ways your prior experiences with power could trip up mutual influence.

Example 1: A Gendered Power Struggle

Matt (42) and Delores (38) are parents of a four-year-old daughter, Maddie. Over the past ten years they successfully created a business together. Delores manages the accounts while Matt is the public face of the company. When Maddie was born, Delores automatically assumed the role of primary caregiver. Growing up with a single-parent mother and absent "deadbeat" father, Maddie witnessed first-hand the effects of gender inequality. She was attracted to Matt's desire for a family and willingness to partner with her in the business. While privately believing that Matt needs her "business head" to make a go of their company, Delores always takes care to credit him for their success. Matt, though cringing at what he calls her "controlling nature," usually goes along with Delores' business plan. Raised in a two-parent household where his father was firmly in charge, he is embarrassed when they and others see Delores appear to be in control.

> What beneath the surface messages about power and influence have Matt and Delores brought to their relationship? How are these related to ideas about gender and family?
>
> _____
> _____
> _____
> _____

How might Delores and Matt's emotional experiences around these messages interfere with mutual influence, despite their success in creating a business?

_____

_____

_____

_____

_____

You may have noticed that Matt and Delores both minimize Delores' contributions to the success of their business. Matt accepts her input, but has mixed feelings about it. On the one hand, accepting her influence violates what he learned about being male and successful; it makes him feel uncomfortable. On the other hand, he has come to depend on her "business head;" he values her input but seldom tells her so. On Delores' part, gratitude that Matt is willing to be a life-partner and socialization to make relationships work make her willing to highlight his positive influence.

However, given the unfair load her mother carried, Delores recognizes unfairness when she sees it. She loves Matt, but is starting to resent his lack of responsiveness to her and Maddie. Delores and Matt are currently in a power struggle in which the more Delores criticizes him for being impervious to her, not influenced by what she and Maddie need, the more passive and disengaged Matt becomes:

DELORES: (*in the morning*) Can you help Maddie get dressed? We're running late.
MATT: (*irritated at the disruption*) I haven't finished my coffee.
DELORES: (*in an accusing tone*) You know I'm supposed to help chaperone Maddie's field trip today. Get off your butt and help for a change!
MATT: Ok. Ok. I forgot. (*Grudgingly heads upstairs.*)
MADDIE: (*ten minutes later*) Mommy, Daddy can't find my shoes.

Delores and Matt are caught in a cycle of negativity in which unequal openness to influence plays a starring role. Their emotional reactions are fueled by their histories with gender and power.

- Matt is not attentive to or influenced by Delores and Maddie's schedules.
- Delores is hurt that Matt does not seem to care enough about her to be open to her needs.
- When Delores criticizes Matt, he feels ashamed for disappointing her but also fears being "controlled" by her.
- Rather than taking steps to change in response to Delores' distress, Matt disengages.
- Delores uses anger to protect herself from additional hurt.
- Matt and Delores never discussed their expectations regarding family, relationship, or business roles.
- Maddie's birth intensified the need for mutual influence and the consequences of the unfairness.

Are any of these responses to influence (or lack of it) familiar to you? How?

_____

_____

_____

_____

_____

Example 2: A Role Reversal?

Alex (49) and Penelope (51) have three teen-aged sons. They are completing this workbook because the joy seems to have gone out of their relationship. They describe themselves as good co-parents, and from the birth of their first child actively took steps to share parenting and household responsibilities. Alex, a graphic designer, organizes his work around child care while Penelope, an obstetrician, "does her part" when she is able to be home. Alex has long wished for more emotional connection with Penelope but justified it based on their hectic schedules. Until Alex raised his concerns, Penelope was "fine" with their relationship. In fact, she counted herself lucky to have a partner that did not put demands on her.

When it comes to intentionally sharing household roles and a relationship based on respect for one another, Alex and Penelope shine. On the surface it even looks like a reversal of stereotypic gender patterns, with Alex accommodating Penelope's high status, demanding job and unpredictable hours. A closer look shows that while Alex is more emotionally influenced by Penelope, their imbalance reflects the consequences of male dominance at the societal level. While completing the activities in this book, Penelope and Alex learned that:

- Alex was raised by a single father who taught him to be sensitive and responsive to the needs of others (which undid stereotypic scripts for men).
- As a result of his loving relationship with his father, Alex is committed to being an involved father and partner in his own family and is more intentional about his roles than many men.
- Penelope was raised in a wealthy family with a "domineering" father who controlled everyone and everything. She witnessed her mother being habitually denigrated and vowed that would never happen to her.
- While in college, Penelope was date-raped. She never told anyone, increased her vigilance in protecting her vulnerability, applied to medical school, and became an advocate for women.
- Penelope married Alex because she believed he would not hurt her. Without realizing it, she continues to protect herself from hurt by maintaining emotional distance.

Are any of these responses to power and influence (or lack of it) familiar to you? How?

_____

_____

_____

_____

_____

We could continue with many different kinds of examples. For example, one partner may almost completely influence the other. This could be because one needs the other a lot more, whether for economic, emotional, or social reasons. These emotional responses are often skewed by societal expectations and standards built into family, gender, and economic roles. For example, men may have learned that they don't (or shouldn't) need relationships. Women may learn to "cover" for them by helping to hide men's dependencies and letting go of their own needs and interests. Often, imbalances in influence are so embedded in your felt social identities (see Chapter 3), that they just seem natural.

Example 3: Unequal Influence in "Shared" Decision-making

Blake (28) and Ramona (27) are three years into their relationship. They need to make a decision about where to live. Ramona has always loved having open space around her; she would rather go a few miles for groceries than have homes packed in close together. Blake grew up in an apartment and values proximity to their favorite eating places. He wants to minimize their impact on the environment by being able to walk or ride a bike. Ramona shares these environmental values but wants to have a small garden and raise some of their food themselves. Then an apartment that Blake particularly likes becomes available:

BLAKE: (*asserts his point of view*) I really like this place. I think we should put in an application right away. It's going to go fast. It's close to all our favorite places and we could each bike to our jobs.

RAMONA: (*attunes to his enthusiasm*) It probably will go fast. You really like it don't you?

BLAKE: (*persists with his perspective*) Yes! I do! We really do need to move fast on this or we'll lose it.

RAMONA: (*hesitates, but doesn't want to disappoint him*) It's not what I was hoping for (*pauses*) but OK. If you're sure…. (*Hopes he'll pick up on her hesitancy.*).

BLAKE: Great! I've got the application right here.

This "shared" decision supports Blake's interests over Ramona's. In fact, "her" decision is based on what she knows Blake wants. Ramona assumed (hoped) Blake understood what she was losing and would take it into account. They are falling into an old, stereotypic gender pattern in which Ramona ends up going along with Blake.

Are any of these responses to power and influence (or lack of it) familiar to you? How?

_____

_____

_____

_____

_____

How Does Influence Work in Your Relationship?

None of the partners in the previous examples *want* influence to be unbalanced. Societal messages and previous histories with power and powerlessness affect what each partner feels, thinks, and does. Once you recognize patterns like these, you can take steps to undo them.

Pause to reflect on how influence works in your relationship(s). Be especially sensitive to ways you may be in a power position. Which of the following areas of influence are at risk of imbalance?

- ❏ Whose topics/interests get discussed
- ❏ Whose schedules organize family/couple routines
- ❏ Whose feelings and interests have an impact on the other
- ❏ Who defines the situation, asserts what's "real"
- ❏ Whose interests are supported in "shared" decisions
- ❏ Who listens, notices, remembers
- ❏ Whose contributions/ideas are minimized or supported
- ❏ Who is likely to automatically accommodate the other
- ❏ Who changes in response to feedback
- ❏ Who is available to the other

What are the barriers to mutual influence in your relationship? When are they most likely to come up?

_____

_____

_____

_____

What is the influence pattern (or patterns) you want to undo? Think of a specific instance as an example.

_____

_____

_____

_____

What will this pattern look like when influence between you and your partner is mutual?

_____

_____

_____

_____

Your Steps to Mutual Influence

Couples that successfully create mutual influence do not rely on what feels natural. They do not just go with the flow or do what feels comfortable. Instead, they take four intentional actions:

1 Center "we"
2 Revise old gender and cultural rules
3 Check in with curiosity about each other
4 Tolerate and learn from conflict

I Center "We"

Your first step to mutual influence is to resist pulls toward individualism. Individualism sets you and your partner(s) in a competitive position in which an equal balance of influence becomes a scorecard of who wins and loses. Even if your give and take is equal, it may not feel relational. When Matt "gave in" to Delores in the first example, he felt controlled by her. Though he accepted her influence, he was not really open to it. It did not come across to Delores as a relational act.

When you take a "we" approach, you emphasize *cooperation*. This is different than simply a compromise in which you each give on something. Cooperation means you and your partner agree on common goals. You work together to support each of you and the relationship overall.

It was not difficult for Matt and Delores to commit to centering "we." When they discussed this step, they agreed that they want to support each other and think in terms of common goals. The going isn't always smooth, but commitment to "we" serves as their touchstone when stressed or irritated.

Return to the pattern of influence you want to undo. Describe the "we" in your new pattern.

_____

_____

_____

_____

What actions on your part will help make this picture real?

_____

_____

_____

_____

What do you know about your partner that may serve as potential common ground upon which to build your "we?"

_____

_____

_____

_____

---

2 Revise Old Gender and Cultural Rules

Within any culture, people do not all live exactly the same. They enact gender and influence in different ways. Your second step is to be more intentional about which cultural rules you want to keep and those you want to revise. In our research (Knudson-Martin & Mahoney, 2009), the only different-gender couples who lived their ideals of mutual influence were those who discussed how they preferred to relate. They revised old models of male dominance and female responsibility for relationships. They didn't always do it perfectly, but they saw themselves on the same team, committed to the relational rules they wanted, and helped each other make them work. Same-gender couples were more likely to do this, since they didn't have historical patterns to automatically follow.

After the one-sided decision about where to live, Ramona is unhappy. She and Blake look back on what happened. They recognize that old gender rules prevented Blake from paying attention to the "we" and told Ramona she should go along with what he wanted. They agree they don't want this to be the pattern for their life together. They decide to rewrite their rules for mutual influence and commit to discussing the long-term consequences of decisions for each of them and their relationship.

What old cultural/gender rules affect the influence pattern(s) you want to change? How?

_____

_____

_____

_____

What new "rule" or guideline would you prefer? Give it words.

_____

_____

_____

_____

What will your new rule look like? What will you be doing? Describe it as if you were narrating a video.

_____

_____

_____

_____

_____

3 Check in with Curiosity About Each Other

The third step is recognizing that when you and your partner are on the same team, you need to know how you're doing. This is a time to be honest and vulnerable. If your partner says something you don't understand or agree with, don't debate (which shuts down openness and learning). Bring your curiosity. Listen. Ask questions grounded in your genuine interest in and care for your partner. Schedule regular times to check-in. Make sure each of you is heard.

If you are in a powerful position (or prone to it because of your place in society), it is especially important that you notice when you may be influencing the topics of the conversation. You may need to take care to stay with (attune to) your partner rather than defending yourself or taking it upon yourself to explain the situation. In the example, when Blake asks Ramona how she likes the new apartment, he does not simply move on when she says, "it's OK." He makes it safe for her to share her unhappiness by being open to her.

Openness to negative feedback and making changes in response is especially important. In fact, failure to be influenced by your partner's negative emotions (anger, disappointment, hurt, etc.) is a major predictor of divorce, especially for men (Gottman, 2011). But positive feedback is also important. Gottman's research found a ratio of five positive messages to one negative is ideal. Expressing only positives doesn't work.

Think about the influence pattern(s) you are trying to change. What do you notice about your partner and how you are influencing her/him/them? What are you curious about?

_____

_____

_____

_____

What do you notice about yourself regarding accepting influence? What would you like your partner to know or understand?

_____

_____

_____

_____

Imagine checking in with your partner on this issue. When could you do it? How would you approach the topic?

_____

_____

_____

_____

How might your influence pattern be different if you and your partner regularly check in with each other? How can you make that happen?

_____

_____

_____

_____

4 Tolerate and Learn from Conflict

Finally, the ability to tolerate and learn from conflict characterizes successful couples. The old gender rules minimized conflict by limiting options for everyone and shutting down female voices. If you have been socialized to "be nice" or put others first, your anger may be a sign of what you have had to suppress. Perhaps like Delores and Penelope in the earlier examples, your anger or efforts to control others are how you protect yourself from additional experiences of powerlessness. Underneath most anger is hurt or fear.

If you are fighting, there are still multiple voices and issues that are important to address. Stopping the fighting without addressing them can be tempting, but creates distance and disappointment. It can also contribute to depression or other signs of distress. An interesting finding from Gottman's (2011) research is that conflict and female expression of anger in the first year of marriage is actually associated with long-term success. Chapter 10 of this book includes strategies for what to do when conflict is especially difficult to discuss.

How do you typically deal with conflict? How is this related to your position of influence in your relationship? To your expectations and experiences around being heard and valued? To your openness (or not) to being influenced by your partner?

_____

_____

_____

_____

_____

_____

What are you learning about yourself and your partner that will help you tolerate and learn from conflict?

_____

_____

_____

_____

What if my partner is not willing to work toward mutual influence or doesn't follow through?

When you approach your partner(s) from your "we" and reach toward their relational interests, they are more likely to open to mutuality. As you put into practice what you are learning, they may experience you as on the same team. You can share how important a supportive back and forth is to you. A therapist may be able to help them get in touch with their relational aspirations. But you cannot create mutual influence by yourself.

What about cultural and religious ideals of male headship?

Cultural and spiritual headship may fit with an orientation toward "we." When it is, this sacred responsibility requires openness to one's partner and family members. The head can best carry out this role when attuned to each person, when he respects and values their knowledge, contributions, and needs. A wise spiritual head centers relationship, is open to influence, and promotes mutual support.

Connecting Through Mutual Influence

Without attunement to your partner and willingness to be vulnerable, receiving influence can result in resentment or feeling controlled. It can seem begrudging or mechanical, as though "checking off a list."

Mutual influence is thus premised on a "we" mindset; it is not simply a behavioral act. Mutual influence grows out of and facilitates connection. It is your signal to each other that you matter. It sustains and embodies love.

Conversation 8

This conversation will help you move toward mutual influence in your relationships. If you are doing it with your partner(s), the conversation sets the stage for your next steps in shared openness to influence. If you are doing it with someone else or on your own, it is an opportunity to evolve what openness to influence means to you. Begin by orienting with openness to yourself and your conversational partners.

Orient with curiosity

- Make yourself comfortable and close your eyes
- Be aware of your breath as it gently goes in and out
- Be aware of any tension, worry, or judgment. Gently let them go
- Open your eyes. Be aware of your conversational partner(s)
- Be aware of the larger world connected to each of you
- Be aware of any tension, worry, or judgment. Gently let them go
- Be aware of your interest in knowing your partner(s)

This activity follows the same conversational structure used in the previous chapters. Each of you responds to the first question for up to two minutes; then you move on to the second and so on. Listeners do not interrupt or comment. When speaking, take time to let your thoughts evolve. Alternate who begins the next question. If you are doing the exercise without a partner, write your answers and then read them aloud to yourself. It is important to hear your voice.

1   Share a story about the feelings that come up for you when you receive or give influence in your relationship(s). What messages from society and your life experience are connected to your feelings? How do they affect you?

2   As you think about mutual influence in your relationship(s), what are you uncertain about or fearful of? What would you like to better understand or know more about? Share an example(s).

3   Share a story about a time when your partner openly received influence from you. What did your partner do? Why was it important to you? What did it say to you about your partner?

4   Share a story about a time when you openly received influence from your partner? What did you do? Why was it important to your partner? What does it say about you?

5   As you and your partner move toward mutual influence, what barriers will you need to overcome? What will the new pattern look like? What will you see? What will you do? What will be meaningful to you?

6　As you listen to your conversational partner(s) today, what moves you? What are you curious about? What thoughts/questions come up? (Partner does not answer.)

7　What would you like your partner to know about your next steps toward mutual influence and tolerating and learning from conflict? About what a "we" position means to you?

Additional Resources

Openness to influence tracker. Use the worksheet in Appendix L to raise awareness about when you are open to influence from your partner and how this affects each of you. You can copy it from the back of the book or download it by visiting www.routledge.com/9781032759890 and clicking on the link that says "Support Material." It is especially helpful if you are in position of power or were socialized to expect you should be in charge or attended to. It can also be helpful for you and your partner to each complete the worksheet and share your observations. Each of you should complete it with openness to learning about your own contributions to mutual influence and what you may want to change. It should not be viewed as a competition.

My emotional map. To better understand your emotions related to influence processes, use the emotional map in Appendix E. You can download www.routledge.com/9781032759890 or print it from the back of the book.

Chapter 9

Share Responsibility for the Relationship

What keeps your relationship going? Who looks out for it, is aware of what is needed to nurture your relational connections, plans for them, and makes sure what is needed gets done? As noted in Chapter 2, this caring work tends to be invisible and underappreciated in society, yet without it relationships wither and die; physical and emotional health suffer.

Sometimes responsibility for relationships is framed as a problem—that you care too much about others. To me, a better question is how is this critical caring work shared? This is both an ethical and practical issue.

In this chapter you will delve into the fourth element of the Circle of Care—the usually hidden world of relational responsibility (figure 9.1). You will address what is involved when each of you does what is necessary to maintain, repair, and enhance your relationship.

What is Relational Responsibility?

You are born entitled to care. You are also obligated to give care. Our ethical responsibility to one another is core to what it means to be part of a community and in relationship. It is not a "tit for tat" sort of exchange where you give this, and in return I give you that. It is responsiveness based on attentiveness to and awareness of one another's unique needs and situations. It is your commitment to the well-being of your partner and to the vitality of the bond between you and to those around you.

Relational responsibility is:

- ongoing and always present
- attentive and proactive to what is needed
- accountable for your impact on others

> Think about the commitment you made (or will make) to your partner. What did this mean to you?
>
> _____
>
> _____
>
> _____
>
> _____
>
> _____

DOI: 10.4324/9781003476528-9

When you made your commitment to your partner, you took it seriously; you wanted to be invested in each other and your life together. You expected your commitment to be mutual. But, as in the other elements of the Circle of Care, there are potential barriers that may limit how you share relational responsibility, including the personal history of care you each bring to your relationships and the societal messages and power contexts that shape your expectations about the giving and receiving of care.

What are Your Expectations About Relational Responsibility?

If you did not receive care that supported your well-being, you may approach new relationships as if "owed to," expecting your partner, children, or others around you to give you the care you did not receive—usually without realizing you are doing so. However, some people who did not receive the care they should have approach relationships with a sense that they are not entitled to care. You may not expect your partner to be there for you and share responsibility for your well-being.

As you think about how you know what to expect regarding reciprocal give and take, consider the messages you received from your family, community, and the larger society.

Example 1: Feels Owed To

Rena sought my help because she was depressed and unhappy. No one in her life seems to meet her expectations—not her husband, not her children, not friends, not even me. Rena describes her parents as emotionally disconnected and more concerned with how their [Jewish] family looked to the [Anglo] community in which they lived. She felt different and lonely at school. When a teacher sexually abused her, Rena did not tell her parents. As an adult Rena has difficulty "being there" for her daughters and is angry and disappointed with her husband. She wants me, her therapist, to see her outside customary hours and more often than usual.

Rena approaches all her relationships with the unconscious hope that others will make up for the deficit of care in her growing up. She is so skewed by her own hurt and pain that she is not able give others the care they deserve. In our work together, we name and validate the injustice she experienced from the abuse and the limited care from her parents and community. Rena, whose grandparents had escaped Nazi Germany, comes to understand her parents' "disengagement" and focus on fitting in as responses to sociopolitical trauma from the Holocaust passed down from generation to generation. This socio-emotional awareness helps Rena develop a more balanced picture of what she is entitled to in relationships and her obligation to also give care and support to others.

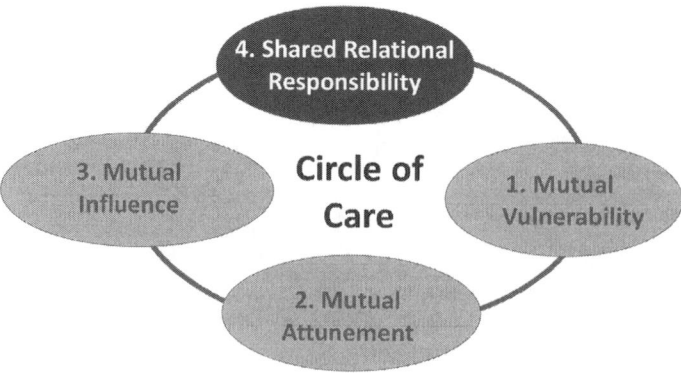

Figure 9.1 Shared relational responsibility—Fourth element in the Circle of Care.

Example 2: Feels Disentitled

Barbara also did not receive the care she was entitled to as a child. But she responded differently.

Barbara came to see me because she is in a new relationship and fears she'll "blow it." She does not have enough money to pay for many therapy sessions, but refuses my offer of a reduced fee. Barbara describes being raised in foster care because her mother "gave her up" when she was five. Her previous two partners are in jail. When we meet with her new partner, Karl, he appears to attune to her and treat her with care and respect. Barbara's challenge is not in being available to give care—which she readily does; it is to expect that she is worthy of love and entitled to receive care.

The Circle of Care gives Barbara a picture of what she has a right to expect in a relationship. It helps her feel comfortable with reciprocity in the balance of caring between her and Karl and to recognize inequities in the relationships with her previous partners. Barbara also comes to see that her mother had not received the care to which she was entitled, and this helps explain (without excusing) the conditions that resulted in her mother's decision to "give her up." She grows more able to appreciate the care she received from her foster parents and open to Karl's care.

More information on Ethics of Care

For more detail about this and the previous case and the contextual model of therapy they illustrate, see Chapter 9 of *Socioculturally Attuned Family Therapy: Guidelines for Equitable Theory and Practice*, 2nd ed. (McDowell et al., 2023).

Example 3: Cultural Expectation to Receive But Not Give

Despite the cultural story that we are "all equal," other societal messages and practices tell you some people are less worthy of care than others, and that some people are expected to give more care than others. For example, women are supposed to give care to men, People of Color are supposed to give care to White people, people with less education and income are expected to care for those with higher status. These unequal expectations affect you at home, at work, and in the broader community.

Zachary came to see me because Abigail, his wife of 20 years, has left him and wants a divorce. He is caught completely by surprise and angry that she has not given him warning. Though no longer interested in working to repair the marriage, Abigail is willing to meet with us to help understand what led to her decision. Abigail says she learned early in their marriage that Zachary expects her to focus on him; when she has other opinions or interests, he gets angry. She has stopped expecting him to attune to and care for her. Though he never hit her, she feels unsafe and on guard. Abigail stayed in the marriage until their son graduated from high school. Now she is leaving.

Zachary never recognized the imbalance in the giving and receiving of care in their marriage. He believed they were each fulfilling their roles as husband and wife—much as his parents had. While he had always loved and appreciated Abigail, Zachary's male socialization did not teach him how to be empathic toward others or focus on their emotional and relational needs. He feels entitled to express anger and other strong emotions without being accountable for his impact on those around him, and depends on Abigail to soothe his emotions. As Zachary becomes aware of the effect of these old gender rules on the people he loves, he is open to learning something new. He does not want to continue to model these cultural scripts for men to his son. The Circle of Care offers him a new way to think about what to expect in a good relationship.

Example 4: Persistence of Gendered Relational Responsibility

Research shows that gendered imbalances in responsibility for caring work are likely to continue even as you move toward equality in other ways.

Ellie and Damon are both university students majoring in computer science. To save money they live with Damon's aunt. In counseling, Ellie describes distress that Damon responded to a request from the aunt by getting up and leaving the room. This leaves Ellie responsible for dealing with his aunt and feeling abandoned by him. When I ask Damon what dealing with his aunt is like for him, he says he is a "geek," that he is not a "people person." Dealing with people makes him nervous.

Damon attributes his behavior to his "nature" rather than gender scripts for men. Once he learns to tune into what his leaving feels like for Ellie, he takes more responsibility for engaging with his aunt and accountability for his effect on Ellie. Discovering that he could overcome his anxiety and doesn't have to limit himself and their relationship to what feels "natural" is an important turning point in their relationship and in Damon's ability to navigate the social world. He realizes that Ellie is also a "geek" who does not easily deal with people (this had been part of their attraction); yet when on auto-pilot he expected her—"the woman"—to carry the relational load. Ellie's insistence on getting help and Damon's openness to learning enables them to discover how to share relational responsibility.

As you read these examples about expectations for care, what thoughts come up for you?

_____

_____

_____

_____

_____

What expectations about the giving and receiving of care have you learned from cultural scripts and your personal and family experiences?

_____

_____

_____

_____

_____

How have these expectations affected you and those around you?

_____

_____

_____

_____

_____

Steps to Sharing Relational Responsibility

There are many aspects of relational responsibility, most of which are not often noticed by others or acknowledged as important. As illustrated in Figure 9.2, sharing relational responsibility first involves raising awareness about the care work in your relationship. Then you can commit to an intentional plan. It also involves responsibility for how you bring yourself into the relationship, monitoring and being accountable for your impact on each other and the relationship, and checking in so that care work does not go back to unnoticed or unappreciated, especially as circumstances and needs evolve over time.

Use the example of Nick and Laurelle to guide your steps toward shared relational responsibility:

Nick and Laurelle have been together since high school, married for 15 years, and have three sons ages 9, 10, and 15. Laurelle works as a home health care provider. Until an injury two years ago, Nick was part of a residential construction crew.

Raise Awareness of Care Work

Use the checklist in Appendix C at the back of the book to raise awareness of the care work that keeps your relationship going and who does it. It identifies five kinds of care work:

1 *Attentiveness to the relationship:* thinking about what others are doing throughout the day and what they need; worrying about their well-being and thinking about them while you are doing something else; thinking about the relationship/family as a whole and what it needs.

Before leaving for work, Laurelle remembers that Taylor (age 15) has a big test today and wishes him well. While at work, Laurelle thinks about the boys' schedules at school and wonders if Brandon (age ten) has been able to focus better in class. When the boys come home from school, Nick tells them to keep the noise down; that they are disturbing him.

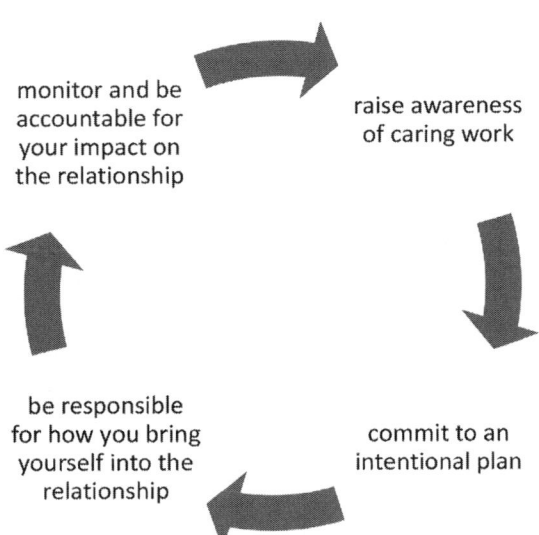

monitor and be accountable for your impact on the relationship

raise awareness of caring work

commit to an intentional plan

be responsible for how you bring yourself into the relationship

Figure 9.2 Steps to shared relational responsibility.

List the ways you were attentive to your partner/family in the last day or two.

_____

_____

_____

2. *Behind the scenes "doing for":* Buying food and other supplies the family needs, picking up after, doing laundry and routine housework, monitoring and attending to health and safety of partner, children, and pets; maintaining communication with extended family and others, and coordinating accomplishment of household tasks and activities.

    Before she leaves for work, Laurelle asks Nick if there is anything he needs her to do for him. On her lunch break she texts Brandon's teacher for an update on his behavior and checks in with her mother. On her way home, she stops to pick up an ingredient for the dinner she has planned. When she arrives home, she asks Nick how he is feeling and asks him to put the basket of laundry in the wash, which he does. She asks Brandon and Logan to help her prepare dinner. After dinner she checks their homework. She asks Nick to join them in watching a movie, which he does.

    List the behind the scenes "doing for" work that you did in the last day or two:

    _____

    _____

    _____

3. *Anticipating and Planning:* maintaining a mental list of everyone's activities and schedules, anticipating what others need and planning social events, arranging childcare, household help, appointments, reminding others of their activities and responsibilities.

    The next morning Laurelle reminds Nick that Taylor has a dentist appointment after school. She says she'll take the bus to work so Nick can use the car to take Taylor to the dentist. On her break at work, she calls a pizza place to arrange for Logan's birthday party. While driving home, she thinks about what Logan might like for his birthday and reminds herself to discuss this with Nick tonight.

    List the anticipating and planning care work you did in the last day or two:

    _____

    _____

    _____

4. *Emotional tending/comfort:* noticing and attending to emotional states of others, helping them process their emotions, showing empathy toward their experience, comforting when down, conceiving of and taking the lead in efforts to support others.

When she comes home from work, Laurelle checks on Brandon and Logan to see how their days went. Brandon is upset because the teacher was "picking on me." Laurelle listens and helps Brandon walk through what happened. She helps him calm his distress, then invites him to help her prepare dinner. After dinner, Nick seems irritable. Laurelle knows he has been struggling with depressed thoughts since being on disability. She focuses on being empathic to his feelings of uselessness and tries to validate how important he still is to her and the boys.

List what you did to emotionally tend or comfort your partner/family in the last day or two.

_____

_____

_____

5. *Managing self-in-relation:* managing your own emotions while working to meet the needs of others, considering the effect of your behavior and decisions on others, making your and relationship needs known, managing how you present your needs and concerns, and calming your own distress to be able to focus on others.

After dinner Nick's back is hurting. Brandon and Logan are poking at each other and making a lot of noise. Nick yells at them to pipe down. When they start up again, he strides into the living room, shuts off the TV and tells them to go to their room. Laurelle is exhausted from her long day and worried about her mother's health. She is irritated that Nick is so hard on the boys, and pauses to take a few breaths to calm herself and put her worries aside. She reminds herself that Nick is in a lot of pain and struggling with self-worth since being on disability, then goes to calm and support him before checking on the boys and their homework.

List what you did to manage your emotions and needs while caring for your partner/family in the last day or two.

_____

_____

_____

In the example, Laurelle is attentive and caring of her partner and children while thinking ahead and planning for their needs. To do so, she has to manage her own emotions. Nick plays a supportive role, and depends on Laurelle to remind him of what needs to be done. He does not try to calm his emotions or manage how he presents his needs to others. No one focuses on Laurelle and her needs.

Review your lists of the caring work you did. How are these important to the well-being of your relationship/family?

_____

_____

_____

_____

_____

What caring work did your partner do? Are there some you might overlook or not be aware of? How are these important to the well-being of your relationship/family?

_____

_____

_____

_____

_____

_____

Commit to an Intentional Plan

What do you need to do to balance how responsibility for your relationship is shared? Because caring work tends to be culturally pre-programed, the caring work done by women or others in less powerful positions tends to be invisible. When men or those in more powerful positions do caring work, it is outside the norm and more likely to be noticed and acknowledged, even when it is not a fair share. It takes an intentional plan to counteract these historical imbalances.

Given the expectations you learned from society and your family/relationships, what do you need to do to create a more equal balance of relational responsibility?

_____

_____

_____

_____

_____

Nick had not realized that he expected Laurelle to smooth the relational waters and plan for them. After talking with Laurelle, he created a list of "thinking about the relationship" and "behind the scenes" work that he commits to doing, for example:

- Check with the boys about school and homework and follow-up with their teachers
- Ask about Laurelle's day and worries about her mother
- Calm myself so anger and irritation do not keep me from "being there" for Laurelle and the boys

*If you learned **not** to focus on your relationship or automatically do the caring work that supports it,* list three actions you will take:

_____

_____

_____

Laurelle had learned to carry the relational weight and not expect others to be there for her. After completing this workbook with Nick, they commit to sharing responsibility for the relationship. Examples of what this means for Laurelle include:

- Be comfortable with Nick and the boys seeing that I am tired or worried
- Work with Nick to create a family calendar and trust his promise to track it
- Draw a line when the imbalance of caring is hurting me or our relationship

If you learned that maintaining relationships rests primarily with you, list three actions you will take:

_____

_____

_____

Your plan for shared relational responsibility will include division of household and domestic tasks, as well as personal accountability for your contributions to the vitality of your relationship and impact on each other. Appendix M at the back of the book provides a guide to help you and your partner create a plan.

A caution about what is fair

Fairness does not necessarily mean you each divide everything 50–50, straight down the middle. You will find the division that works best for you. But—our research found that most couples got stuck in an unequal balance because each did what they felt comfortable with or already had skills for. These are often gendered or taken-for-granted; i.e., she is better at changing diapers or dealing with emotions. Real change may require learning something new. Laurelle has to resist the temptation to take over when Nick tries to help Brandon with his homework. Nick has to recognize and focus on relational matters he did not think about before.

Check-in Together

You are changing old patterns that persistently catch modern couples. You are in this together. It is not a contest or competition. Set a time to check in with each other about how it is going. Learn from one another and keep your relational goals at the forefront.

Be Responsible for How You Bring Yourself into the Relationship

An agreement about who will do what when helps keep old patterns from re-emerging, but it is not enough. You must each also take responsibility for what you bring to the relationship and how you engage. Three principles are helpful:

- Know yourself
- Stay present
- Be honest

Know Yourself

When you understand how your place in the world and personal experiences have influenced what you expect and do, you are more able to see what you bring to your relationships and make adjustments to help you reach your relational goals. Nick realizes he reacted to his injury by disengaging from Laurelle and the family; that anger and feeling useless were responses to societal messages that measured his worth by his ability to be "productive" and created expectations that others would manage his emotions. He decides to engage instead. Similarly, when Laurelle sees that she learned to keep her needs to herself and not bother others with them, she is able to change her expectations.

What do you know about yourself and your place in the world that affects what you bring to your relationships?

_____

_____

_____

_____

Stay present

When there is conflict or you feel hurt, afraid, or resentful, it is easy to disengage—to emotionally shut down, use anger to create a barrier, or physically distance yourself. This can sometimes keep things smooth in the short term, but increases distance and disappointment over time. Ask yourself what you need to do to stay present, as well as make it safe for your partner to stay present. If you need a little space or time, ask for it in a way that maintains connection to your partner. When anger pops up, Nick now breaths to calm himself and reminds himself to go toward his relationships. Laurelle resists emotionally shutting down and brings her full self to the relationship, previously hidden resentments as well as love.

What do you need to do to stay physically and emotionally present in your relationship?

_____

_____

_____

_____

Be honest

You can be honest without being hurtful. When speaking from your experience, your partner can know you. Sometimes you may not know what is going on for you. Be honest about that. Use the emotional map in Appendix E to sort out what you are experiencing. For example, Laurelle likes to connect with the boys about school and their lives. She also feels resentful that Nick seems to leave all this to her and is sad for the boys that their dad does not seem interested in them. She is honest about this with Nick:

LAURELLE: I love checking in with the boys about school and what is going on for them. But it feels unfair that I do almost all of this—and that I am always the one to talk to their teachers. It would be better if we could share this load. I think it will be better for the boys too.

When Laurelle says she does most of the checking in with the boys, Nick feels shame and a desire to defend himself. He takes a breath to stay present. As he acknowledges her statement, he realizes that he used to engage with the boys by wrestling with them and playing basketball, but his injury prevents that. And, he never felt comfortable communicating with the school or helping with homework. He is honest about the unfairness and about his uncertainty:

NICK: (*takes another deep breath*) You are right. You do almost all of the checking on homework and talking with the teachers. I feel bad that I can't wrestle and shoot hoops with the boys like I used to. (*Thinks a moment.*) School was never easy for me. I don't feel very competent about helping them.

Until Nick and Laurelle talked about it and brought the unfairness out of the shadows, it was "natural" for Laurelle to take on this responsibility. Talking honestly about it made it possible to address the unfairness; for Nick to step out of his comfort zone without feeling that Laurelle was attacking him, and for Laurelle to share this load without having to give up the closeness she feels with the boys.

What do you need to do to be honest in your relationships? About what?

_____

_____

_____

_____

Monitor and Be Accountable for Your Impact on the Relationship

Finally, relational responsibility involves paying attention to how what you do and say and the choices you make affect your partner and others around you. Your attunement skills (Chapter 7) will help you notice and think about your impact on them. Your willingness to be vulnerable (Chapter 6) will help you be accountable for hurts you may have caused and to take initiative in re-building your connection when it is [temporarily] torn.

Even in times when the need for care is not equal (for example, if one of you is sick or going through a crisis), each of you needs to be able to give as well as receive, to monitor and be accountable for your impact on each other and the relationship. Nick discovered that when he is accountable for how he affects Laurelle and the boys and makes changes to share relational responsibility, he feels better physically and emotionally as well.

Connecting Around Shared Relational Responsibility

This conversation will help you bring caring work out of the background. It is an opportunity to recognize and appreciate the importance of this labor and to be accountable for your contributions. If you are doing the conversation with your partner, you can talk directly about what shared relational responsibility will look like in your relationship. If you are doing it with others or on your own, you can envision what shared relational responsibility will look like.

Conversation 9

Begin by orienting to your conversational partner(s) with curiosity and openness to learning.

Orient with curiosity

- Make yourself comfortable and close your eyes
- Be aware of your breath as it gently goes in and out
- Be aware of any tension, worry, or judgment. Gently let them go
- Open your eyes. Be aware of your conversational partner(s)
- Be aware of the larger world connected to each of you
- Be aware of any tension, worry, or judgment. Gently let them go
- Be aware of your interest in knowing your partner(s)

As in previous chapters, each of you responds to the first question for up to two minutes; then you move on to the second and so on. Listeners do not interrupt or comment. When speaking, take time to let your thoughts evolve. Alternate who begins the next question. If you are doing the exercise without a partner, write your answers and then read them aloud to yourself. It is important to hear your voice.

1   Tell a story about a time when relational responsibility was shared? How did you know? What is important to you about this story?

2   Tell a story about a time when relational responsibility was not shared? What was your part in the imbalance? How did the imbalance affect you? How did it affect your partner/others?

3   When you think about your responsibility to your partner, what societal messages and life experiences influence your expectations? Share some examples. How do these expectations affect the balance of relational responsibility?

4   When you think about what you need to do to more fairly share caring work in your relationship, what questions come up for you? What are you uncertain about? Give examples.

5   When relational responsibility (caring work) is shared in your relationship, how will you know? What will you see. Describe it as though narrating a video of what happens, who does what. What is important to you about this picture?

6   As you listen to your conversational partner's responses, what is meaningful to you? What new thoughts or questions come up? How do these affect you? (Partner does not answer.)

7   What specific commitments to sharing responsibility for maintaining your relationship are you able/willing to make? Why are these important to the quality of your relationship? Why are they important to you?

Additional Resources

Our plan to share responsibility for the relationship. To guide how you and your partner agree to share caring work and responsibility for the relationship, copy Appendix M from the back of the book or download it by visiting www.routledge.com/9781032759890 and clicking on the link that says "Support Material." It will help you detail the pieces that need to be done to sustain a relationship on a day-by-day, practical basis and provides space to record your plan and commitment to each other. It also invites you to decide how you will check in with each other to evaluate how sharing responsibility for the relationship is going and what you may need to change.

Another guide to fairness. Eve Rodsky (2019) wrote *Fair Play: Share the Mental Load, Rebalance Your Relationship, and Transform Your Life.* It offers concrete strategies for sharing the mental and physical work of running a family. Many couples find it helpful.

Chapter 10

Oh No! Not Again

Persistently Return to Your Relational Goals

Do not be surprised when an old socio-emotional habit seems to persist. It can take time to solidify your evolving relational map. And, disagreements are normal. Successful couples are distinguished by how they respond. In this chapter you will learn how to solidify change and what to do when problems return.

How to Sustain Change

Change happens as you live it. New ideas and experiences need to become embodied—to literally become part of you and your relationships. Old socio-emotional stories that defined you and limited your relationships are replaced by new ones. This is a bit like brain surgery or gardening. You create the neural and relational pathways you nurture, prune or weed out blocks to your shared growth and health, and provide a supportive environment. Four practices are key:

- Orient to "we"
- Look for and expand what works
- Learn from negatives
- Develop a supportive community

> **What relational changes are you trying to make? What will you see when the changes are real?**
>
> _____
> _____
> _____
> _____
> _____
> _____
> _____

Orient to "We"

Whether coping with stress, illness, or even stopping smoking, most successful change takes a "we" approach. In her study of committed couples who thrive, psychologist Karen Skerrett (2022) heard the same words over and over, "we are in this together."

Think about your life and the changes you are making as something you are in together. If this is not yet automatic, create ways to put yourselves in touch with your commitment to "we" and to the "we" you are becoming. In the example below, Omar is intentional in framing a decision about a personal activity in terms of their "we."

DOI: 10.4324/9781003476528-10

Example: Use "We/Our" Language

Omar's friends approach him about getting season tickets for their favorite football team. In the past, Omar would have said "yes," and then told Tatiana. Now, he reminds himself to consider the expense and time commitment in terms of his relationship with Tatiana. He uses "our" and "we" in his response to his friends: "Tatiana and I need to check our budget and schedule; I'll get back to you soon." He uses a similar mindset when he approaches Tatiana, "[Friends] asked me to go in with them on season tickets for the [football team]. We haven't talked about our plans for the fall; how would this work for our budget and time together?"

Tangible reminders of your connection and commitment, such as "Our Picture of We" (Appendix N), help keep "we" at the forefront. When disruption or disconnection arise, Tatiana and Omar pause to remind themselves, "We'll find a way through." They also orient to "be with" when one of them is dealing with a personal transition or struggle.

Example: Shared Coping

After a long day, Tatiana picks up the children from daycare, but has a headache and is having a hard time being patient. She is pulling double-duty at work because a colleague is on maternity leave and a fill-in has not been found. When she gets home, Omar has dinner nearly ready and steps in to take charge of the children so she can rest. Tatiana and Omar see her extra workload as a shared problem. They decided she will continue to pick up the children because the daycare is close to her work, but Omar will take the lead in planning dinner and cooking.

Look For and Expand What Works

Even when old patterns persist, there are times when they do not. Other times, your change is not as perfect or complete as you would like, but part of it is there. Distressed couples are likely to emphasize what is not yet working. You will be more successful when you look for times when you or your partner has made the change you are seeking or have taken a small step toward it. Notice it. Name it. Then ask yourself or each other what you did to make this possible? **And do it again.** Acknowledge the positive consequences. Then you can consider what the next small step toward your goal will look like and work toward that.

To repeat:

- Notice what works (even though small or incomplete)
- Acknowledge positive consequences
- Ask what made this possible
- Do it again
- Take the next small step

Example: Noticing What Works

Tatiana and Omar are working toward mutual vulnerability. Omar knows he struggles with accepting help and admitting mistakes. Tatiana has learned that she tends to "protect" Omar by holding back input or concerns that might disturb him. Tonight, as they are getting the children ready for bed, each does something a little different. When Omar starts to engage their young son, Kai, in a lively song, Tatiana says, "That song gets Kai real excited. It's better to save it for another time and pick a quieter song to help him sleep." Omar pauses a moment and says, "You're right—silly of me" and moves into a quieter song. A little later they process what happened:

TATIANA: Thanks for taking my suggestion about a quieter song. It helped me feel like we are parenting as a team, and that you appreciate my input.

OMAR: Yeah. It felt good to me too. And it got Kai to settle down.

TATIANA: What do think made this work so well? What helped you be open to my suggestion?

OMAR: I think I was just focused on getting Kai to sleep. (*Pauses to reflect.*). And those ideas that a man always has to look competent didn't come up.

As they discuss it a little more, they decide that seeing themselves as part of a team helped each of them risk vulnerability. They agree to try it again.

What is something you did recently that demonstrated the relational change you are seeking (or moved a little closer to it)? What did you do to make this possible?

_____

_____

_____

_____

What is something your partner did recently that demonstrated the relational change you are seeking (or moved a little closer to it)? What did he/she/they do to make this possible?

_____

_____

_____

_____

_____

Learn from Negatives

Blow-ups happen. A return to an old pattern when things have been going better can feel especially hurtful or disillusioning. It's easy to think you are back to square one. But you are not. Discord and disappointment are normal steps on the path to a more satisfying and loving relationship. Sometimes it is a sign that the person whose voice had been stifled in the old patterns is now more comfortable to speak. Sometimes it is a signal that you have been making important changes but have issues you were previously not aware of or avoided. It is often a sign that old societal messages can still reach in and take hold.

When this happens:

- Avoid escalation
- Take a breath (or a few)
- Focus on what happened before you try to find a solution
- Listen with curiosity and openness to understanding
- Apply and update your socio-emotional awareness (see Chapter 3)
- Identify what you learned (about yourself, your partner, your relationship)
- Return to "we" to find your path forward

Example: Learning from Negativity

Tatiana is looking forward to a celebratory party at the home of one of her best friends. The babysitter has arrived, she has on the outfit purchased for the occasion. But Omar is nowhere to be seen. When she calls him, he says he is working late on a project and that she should go by herself. Tatiana goes to the party, but is hurt that Omar is "blowing off" something important to her. When people ask where Omar is, she starts to tear up. She can't enjoy the party and leaves early. When Omar gets home, she shouts at him in anger and then dissolves into tears. Omar feels bad, but thinks she is blowing this out of proportion. He hardly knows the couple hosting the party.

After some back-and-forth anger, Omar takes a deep breath and avoids further escalating the situation, "I'm sorry. Can we talk about how this happened?" It takes Tatiana a few minutes to be open to conversation, but Omar gives her time. Tatiana describes how she had been looking forward to doing something special together and that she wanted Omar and her friends to know each other. Instead of pressuring her to "let it go" (and make him feel better—the old pattern) or blaming her for not being clearer about why the party was important to her, he listens and tries to understand. Omar realizes he has been focused on "doing his share" around the house, but not really attuned to her. And sometimes old messages tell him a man should have more autonomy— more freedom.

As they explore what happened, Tatiana feels heard and reminds them that changing old sociocultural patterns is challenging, that they are "in this together." Going forward, they agree to focus on attunement and time together, not just getting the work done. They also agree to be honest about what they are feeling.

Reflect on a time when something negative happened in your relationship? What can you learn about yourself from this incident? How is this understanding helpful to your relationship?

_____

_____

_____

_____

_____

_____

As you reflect on this incident, what would you like to know more about from your partner's perspective? How might this understanding be helpful to your relationship?

_____

_____

_____

_____

_____

Develop a Supportive Community

Positive change is more likely to hold when you speak about it and share your positive vision with others. You will continue to receive many individualistic messages from the larger society that work against your relationship (see Chapter 2). You need people around you who share your relational values. This moves change from something purely personal and fragile to something stronger, held among you and a supportive community.

To expand your process of change beyond you and your partner:

- Tell people what you are learning about how to nurture mutually supportive relationships
- Identify people who support your relationship and spend time with them
- Get involved in advocacy and activities that promote equity and relational values

Example: Making relational goals public

After their discussion about the party, Omar and Tatiana realize they have been alone with their changes. They have friends individually, but have not developed friendships that see them as a couple and support their movement toward shared relational responsibility. They decide to make their relational goals public and to build community with others who share them.

Omar is having a beer with his buddies and says he has to go home because he told Tatiana he would be back in time to put the kids to bed. One of his friends laughs and says, "She's got a chain around you, Man!" Instead of laughing back, Omar responds with a new message about relationships, "No. Tatiana and I are a team. She's making my life richer, not tying me down." He's surprised when another friend jumps in to support his [new] message about relationships, "[to friend] Yeah, Bud. You might be doing better with [his girlfriend] if you paid more attention to her!" It feels risky to resist out loud the old cultural message that relationships restrict men's freedom. But when Omar does, he opens a new conversation about masculinity and relationships—and finds he is not alone.

Tatiana and Omar also begin developing shared relationships. Over pizza with friends, they talk about this workbook and how they are using it to build a more mutually supportive relationship. Soon everyone is talking, because they are all dealing with similar issues. They decide to have monthly "SERT (Socio-Emotional Relationship Therapy) and Snacks" gatherings in which they focus on what works to build relationships—what they are learning or thinking about as they center "we." They also begin to discuss how they can help children in the community learn that relational principles are not just for girls.

In the example, Omar and Tatiana's change is solidified as they engage with others to develop and expand upon a shared image of what reciprocally responsive relationships look like in real life. This new relational story in not just personal, it is societal. Their focus on what works moves beyond a negative story that pits partners and individual needs against each other to a vision of mutually supportive relationships that promote health and enable creative responses to life's challenges.

A word of caution

While awareness of the gap between your ideals of mutual support and what most couples actually do is important, focusing primarily on the problem will not create much change. If all you and your friends do is complain to each other, your friendship and family communities are likely to promote negativity toward your relationship rather than actions to change it. When you notice a preponderance of this kind of conversation, shift the topic to how you will know when your relationship is more equitable and mutually supportive, what you will see. This will help you and your friends/family begin to develop an image of what to move toward and how to recognize small steps. And, shift the topic to what works, what you did that spurred a change toward shared relational responsibility or expanded a small one.

Who in your life supports your evolving relationship?

_____

_____

_____

What do you (or could you) share with others about the relational changes you are making?

_____

_____

_____

_____

How will your story about what it means to be in a mutually supportive relationship be different when you share this ideal with others and discuss what works?

_____

_____

_____

_____

What kinds of changes in your community would help expand the culture to include a picture of what mutually supportive relationships look like and why they are important? What could you do to help promote this idea?

_____

_____

_____

_____

BEST Conversations for Difficult Topics

There may be things about which you and your partner will never agree and need to cooperate. There may be highly charged topics that snag you emotionally and are hard to address. Some issues may sit like a cloud above you. You know they are there, but dealing with them brings a sense of foreboding so you avoid them. Happy, loving couples who otherwise mutually support each other are likely to face these difficult topics from time to time. They are a part of sharing a life together with more than one voice and set of experiences.

Example: A standoff

Tatiana and Omar avoid talking about his mother (Eva). Every time they do, they end up in an argument or standoff. Tatiana thinks Eva is too harsh and judgmental. She thinks Eva is not a good influence on the *children and tries to avoid leaving Eva alone with them. Omar wants his mother to be able to spend more time with the children, as she would like to do.*

BEST conversations provide a format for dealing with difficult topics. Like the conversations you've been having as you go through this book, you set aside debate and postpone search for an answer. You begin with openness to learning about yourself and each other. The structured format gives each of you space to listen and space to be heard. You are able to see each other and the topic from multiple angles and reflect on possibilities and make an agreement about whatever comes next, with trust that you will work through challenges as they arise. Four phases (BEST) are involved (see Figure 10.1):

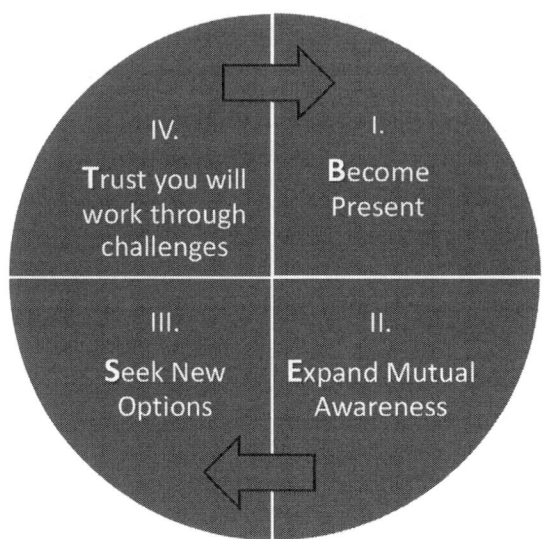

Figure 10.1 Phases of BEST conversations.

1 Become Present

BEST conversations are planned. You and your partner set aside time to focus on a topic that troubles you. Before jumping into the subject, each of you reviews your **emotion map** as it relates to this topic (Appendix E) and **brings a copy** to the conversation. You take time to quiet yourselves, feel centered within a web of relationships, apply socio-emotional awareness to your reactions (Chapter 3), and be present to your partner and to the issue.

The following steps enable you to be present:

A. Agree on an amount of time for getting in touch with yourselves and becoming present. Take at least five minutes.

B. Silently review your emotion maps (Appendix E) as they relate to the topic you are about to discuss.

C. Close your eyes, make yourself comfortable, and take slow, deep breathes in…and out…

D. As you continue to gently breathe in and out, picture yourself within expanding circles of relationships. Be aware of your partner… your places of belonging… how you know yourself in the world.

E. As you breathe in and out, let yourself be present to the topic for discussion. Be aware of tensions you feel around this subject… where you feel them in your body… what shoulds/oughts or right/wrongs are present… what these say about you and what matters to you.

F. As you continue to gently breathe in and out, let these tensions relax. Let them "be." Be aware of your partner and your interest in their perspectives… in what matters to them.

G. As you continue to slowly breathe in and out, orient yourself to learning with curiosity and openness to new awareness and possibilities.

Example: Being present and open

As Tatiana reflects on her emotion map, she is aware of a strong urge to protect her children, along with fears that she is not a good mother. As she expands her circle beyond Omar and her close friends, she is aware that as a 1.5-generation immigrant (born in another country but grew up in the US), she often feels judged in the larger society. As she breathes in and out, she relaxes and lets herself get in touch with her desire to understand Omar and be present with him. Similarly, as Omar focuses inwardly, he is aware that he feels protective of his mother and anxious about upsetting Tatiana. As he breathes in and out, he feels the pressure begin to release and opens himself to the conversation.

2 Expand Mutual Awareness

In this phase your goal is to understand the multiple facets of your reactions to this issue and learn about those of your partner. Both the structure for communicating and the order of the questions are important.
   Faithfully follow these guidelines:

- Each of you responds to the first question for two minutes. When you are talking, take time to let your thinking evolve but do not speak longer than two minutes.
- When one of you is speaking, the other(s) does **not interrupt or comment**. When you are listening, focus on your partner. Resist the urge to [even silently] question, add, disagree, etc.
- Move on to the next question, repeating the format.

How you communicate is more important than the eventual solution or agreement. When the impulse to directly answer or debate each other arises, gently and respectfully remind yourselves to return to the structured process.

Awareness Questions

1   Share a story that shows why [this topic] is important to you. The story (or stories) may be from any time and place in your life. Explain what about this story is meaningful to you.

2   What messages related to your felt identities (gender, race/ethnicity, class, sexuality, abilities, etc.) come up around [this topic]? What do they say you *should* think, feel, or do? Where do these messages come from?

3   When [this topic] comes up between you, what is your fear or worry? How do you experience this fear? What does it say about you and/or the situation? Use your emotion map as a guide.

4   When [this topic] comes up between you, what is your hope or dream? What does this dream mean to you? Use your emotion map as a guide.

5   What are you uncertain or confused about regarding [this topic]? What are you flexible about? Explain.

6   As you listen to your own and your partner's responses to these questions, what new awareness, ideas, or questions come up for you? What would you like to know more about? (Partner does not answer.)

7   What will it mean to you when [this topic] brings less trouble or division between you? What will it say about your relationship? About you? About you partner? Explain.

After completing these questions, it can be helpful to go back to the first question and repeat the sequence again following the same format. The second round enables you to build upon and expand beyond your initial responses, which adds new layers of understanding. You may also repeat this format on other days or when the topic emerges again.

Example: New awareness

Tatiana and Omar have always been so focused on whether or not Eva will spend time with the children that they never really heard each other on this topic. They did not even fully understand their own reactions. As they reflect on and respond to these questions, Tatiana begins to see how much Omar values his mother—and her own role as a mother. Each begins to see their "problem" in relation to their different sociocultural experiences and fears. Omar had not realized Tatiana felt judged in the larger society (and by his mother). Each concluded that finding a positive way for Eva to be involved with the children was important.

3 Seek New Options

In this phase you brainstorm how to proceed. Since previous efforts left this subject unresolved or a sore spot, now is the time to be creative, to try something new. What you each previously thought the other should do probably won't work. Instead, you choose how to cooperate.

Approach the seeking options phase with:

*   open minds
*   a sense of playful togetherness
*   respect for multiple voices
*   a back-and-forth flow of ideas
*   attention to equity and fairness

There are three steps:

(A)   Brainstorm. Let ideas flow with minimum discussion. Use Appendix Q to record your thoughts and ideas. It has three "pots" for your thoughts and ideas.

> Pot 1—list take-aways from your previous conversation
> Pot 2—list possible agreements/solutions—no matter how silly they may seem
> Pot 3—list small changes that could matter

Make additions to any of these lists as you think of them:

(B)   Discuss and organize your brainstormed lists.

*   What jumps out at you?
*   Where is there overlap?
*   What is new that you didn't see before?
*   Explore how specific possibilities might work
*   Don't rush to agreement—leave room to discuss without commitment

(C)   Make a temporary agreement.

Agree to cooperate on something. It could be as simple as agreeing to disagree, a small first step that each of you are willing to take, or a new shared vision of what cooperation around this issue looks like.

Example: Agreement to small steps

*Creating the "three pots" of ideas takes the debate and pressure off Tatiana and Omar. They begin to feel like they are approaching the problem together. The list of small steps is especially helpful. They find there are many. They agree on two small steps to get started—Omar will take his mother to lunch with the goal of letting her know how much he values her **and** how much he values Tatiana, especially as a mother. Tatiana will ask Eva to pick the children up from day care one day soon. While Eva gives the children dinner and gets them ready for bed, Tatiana and Omar will go out. They will evaluate in two weeks and go from there.*

4 Trust You Will Work Through Challenges

The final step of your BEST conversation is trust that you and your partner(s) will continue to evolve understanding and cooperation on this issue. You expect that new challenges will arise. Your commitment to each other is to work through them together. This involves commitment to relationality, equity, and mutual support through the Circle of Care and recognition that developing socio-emotional awareness is a lifelong process that evolves as you and your circumstances change.

Example: Commitment to keep the conversation going

Tatiana and Omar don't know how their initial steps to engage Eva in their children's lives will work. They agree to keep the conversation going to work out this problem and to address new ones as they arise.

Describe your commitment to work through challenges:

_____

_____

_____

_____

_____

When to Get Help

Working with a couple therapist/counselor can help you attain the reciprocally responsive, mutually supportive relationships you want. This option is important when:

- You need additional support to develop the relational practices this book describes
- Your partner has not been willing or able to complete this book with you
- Other issues such as alcohol and substance use, prior physical, sexual, or emotional abuse, experiences of trauma or loss, or struggles with mental health complicate your relationship

Look for a licensed marriage and family therapist, psychologist, psychiatrist, counselor, or social worker who **specializes in relationships**. Seek someone who works from a systems/relational perspective and emphasizes work with gender, culture, and power/control issues and/or the impact of the larger social world on personal and relational well-being.

The following organizations maintain lists of licensed professionals who specialize in relationship work:

- The American Association for Marital and Family Therapy www.aamft.org/Directories/Find_a_Therapist.aspx
- The American Family Therapy Academy https://www.afta.org/find-a-therapist#/

Example: Regular relationship check-ups

Omar and Tatiana visit with a relationship therapist to help them notice and be accountable for their impact on each other. They want help recognizing how their varying cultural histories and socio-emotional identities affect their responses in the Circle of Care. They decide to periodically check in with their therapist when faced with new stresses and transitions, much like they utilize the guidance of other health care professionals.

Creating and Maintaining the Relationship You Want

Each chapter of this book has helped you know what a loving, mutually responsive and supportive relationship looks like. You have taken steps to move toward this relational ideal and expect to return to this guide as you evolve your relationships and/or develop new ones. The final conversation helps you reflect on what you are learning and how to apply it.

Conversation 10

Begin by orienting to your conversational partner(s) with curiosity and openness to learning.

Orient with curiosity

- Make yourself comfortable and close your eyes
- Be aware of your breath as it gently goes in and out
- Be aware of any tension, worry, or judgment. Gently let them go
- Open your eyes. Be aware of your conversational partner(s)
- Be aware of the larger world connected to each of you
- Be aware of any tension, worry, or judgment. Gently let them go
- Be aware of your interest in knowing your partner(s)

As in previous chapters, each of you responds to the first question for up to two minutes; then you move on to the second and so on. Listeners do not interrupt or comment. When speaking, take time to let your thoughts evolve. Alternate who begins the next question. If you are doing the exercise without a partner, write your answers and then read them aloud to yourself. It is important to hear your voice.

1   Share a story that exemplifies what is important to you about the lessons in this book. Why is this story important to you now?

2   Describe a moment when you were touched by something your conversational partner(s) said or did or by the examples in this book. What is meaningful to you about this moment?

3   When you think back on this book a few years from now, what will stand out to you? How will this have affected you? Describe what you will see or do.

4   When you think about your place in the world and how you know yourself and others, what stands out to you? How will this be important to you and the quality of your relationships? Describe what you will see or do.

5   When you think about mutuality in the Circle of Care, what stands out to you? How is this important to the future of your relationships? Describe what you will see or do.

6   When you think about closing the gap between the relationship you want and the relationship you have, what are you uncertain about? What are you wondering about? What do you need to learn/understand?

7   As you listen to your conversational partner(s) today, what new ideas or questions arise for you? What would you like to know more about? How are these important to you? (Partner does not answer.)

8   As you complete this step on your journey to loving, mutually supportive relationships, what commitment are you taking forward? How will this commitment affect you and your relationships?

Additional Resources

Our Picture of "We." Create a picture that represents your "we." As you work together on it, discuss the values you want to live by, what characterizes the "we" you are together. Frame it and place where you can see it. For guidance on this project, copy Appendix N from the back of the book or download it by visiting www.routledge.com/9781032759890 and clicking on the link that says "Support Material."

Another way to create your picture of "we" is to use shadow boxes to make an altar to express what is meaningful to you as a couple. *Altares*, as they are called in Spanish, are especially significant in Latino, Indigenous, Catholic, and Afro-Caribbean cultures as a way to publicly honor important relationships (see Bermúdez & Bermúdez, 2002).

SERT group reflections. The *Socio-Emotional Relationship Workbook for Couples* is ideal for use in groups. Copy or download Appendix O for guidelines on how groups can use reflecting processes to take in the perspectives of others and expand awareness, while avoiding debate and judgment. They may be applied in a variety of group formats.

BEST Format Summary. Appendix P provides a summary of the BEST format for discussing difficult topics with questions for each phase of the conversation. Copy or download and print it as a handy guide.

BEST Brainstorming Record. Copy or download and print the form in Appendix Q to record your brain storming ideas. Putting your collective ideas in front of you on one form makes it easier for you and your partner to seek a temporary agreement together rather than approach the process as an argument.

Appendix A: The Relational You

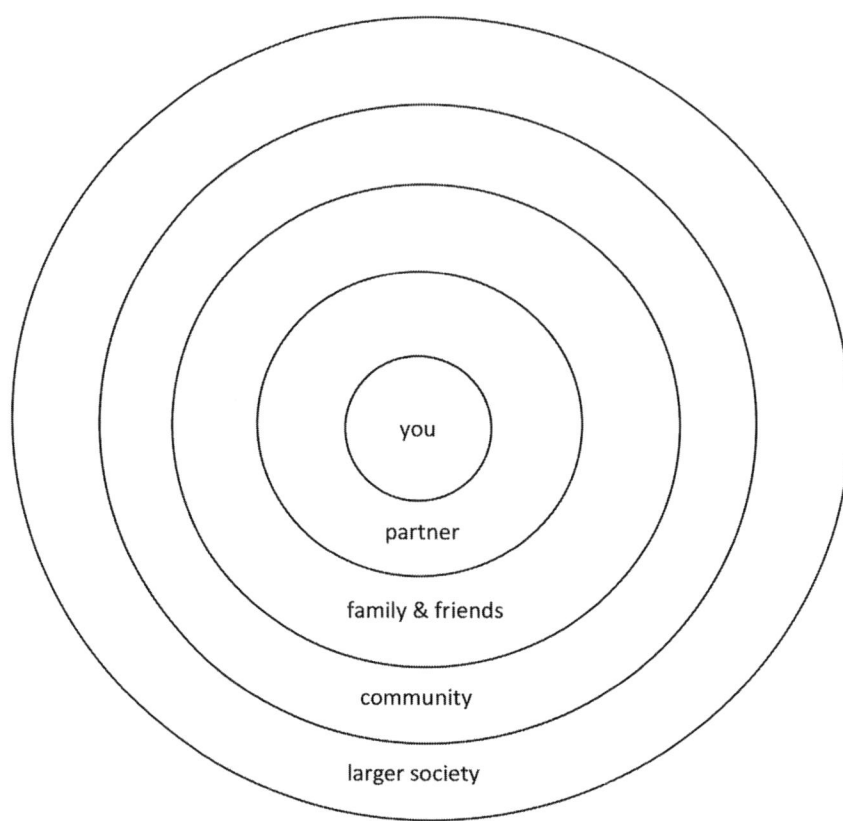

In the spaces between the circles, write the names of specific people and groups in your world. For community include workplace, school, church, other associations, as well as the racial/ethnic and social class groups to which you identify. For the larger society consider wider social forces such as capitalism, patriarchy, democracy, heteronormativity, and dominant cultural value systems such as Euro-American. You can also complete one diagram from when you were a child and compare with your partner.

As you complete this diagram of your relational world, what thoughts or feelings come up for you?

What is it like to see yourself and your relationships within this wider lens?

Appendix B: The Circle of Care

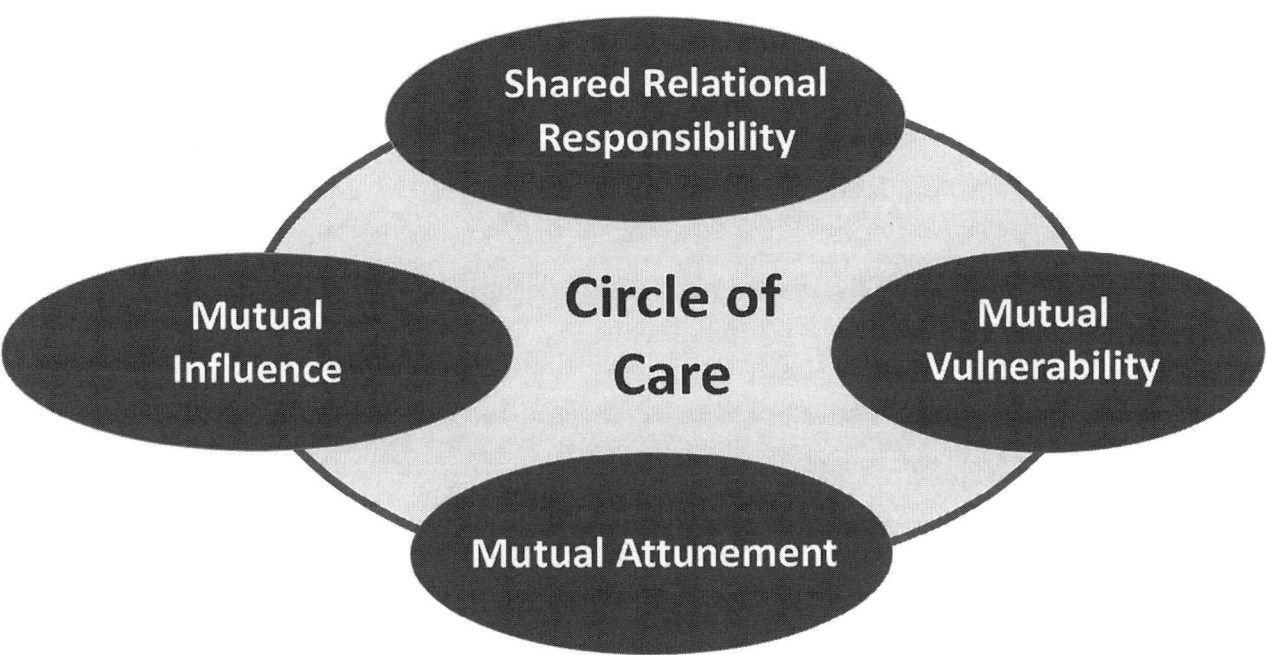

Our commitment to mutual support (write in your words)

Appendix C: Care Work Checklist

Use this list as a guide for conversation about "care work." For each item consider:

1 How is this care work important and helpful?
2 Who in our relationship does this work?
3 How can this care work be more balanced in our relationship/family?

Attentiveness to relationship

❑ Thinking about how partner/others are doing and what they need
❑ Being mindful of what partner/others are doing throughout the day
❑ Worrying about partner's/other's well-being
❑ Thinking about partner's/child's/other's experience while doing something else
❑ Thinking about how the relationship/family as a whole is doing and what it needs

Behind the scenes "doing for"

❑ Buying food, grooming and household supplies that partner/family needs
❑ Picking up after, doing laundry, attending to routine housework by default
❑ Monitoring and attending to the health and safety of partner, children, pets
❑ Maintaining communication with extended families and others
❑ Coordinating accomplishment of household tasks and activities

Anticipating & planning

❑ Maintaining a mental list of partner's and children's activities and schedules
❑ Worrying about and anticipating what others need
❑ Planning social events with family/extended family/friends
❑ Arranging childcare, household help, appointments for health care, etc.
❑ Reminding partner/others of their activities and responsibilities

Emotional tending/comfort

❑ Noticing, monitoring, and attending to partner's/family member's emotional states
❑ Helping partner/family members process their emotions
❑ Showing empathy toward partner's/family member's experiences
❑ Comforting partner/child/others when they are "down"
❑ Conceiving of and taking the lead in efforts to support partner/child/others

Managing self-in-relation

❑ Managing own emotions while working to meet needs of others
❑ Considering the effect of own behavior and decisions on partner/family/relationship
❑ Making own and relationship needs evident to/for your partner
❑ Managing how you present your own needs and concerns to partner/others
❑ Calming your own distress to be able to focus on other

Appendix D: Socio-Emotional Awareness Log

What happened? What I felt, thought, or did.	What societal ideas related to my felt identities were activated? (biological sex and gender identity; race and ethnicity; economic and education level; sexual orientation; culture and religion; body and abilities; family structure, migration and legal statuses; other relevant identities)	How did this affect my relationship? How do I prefer to respond?

Appendix E: My Emotional Map

Use this map to increase your personal emotional awareness of a situation. Begin with your bodily sensations and emotional state and move outward toward the other circles

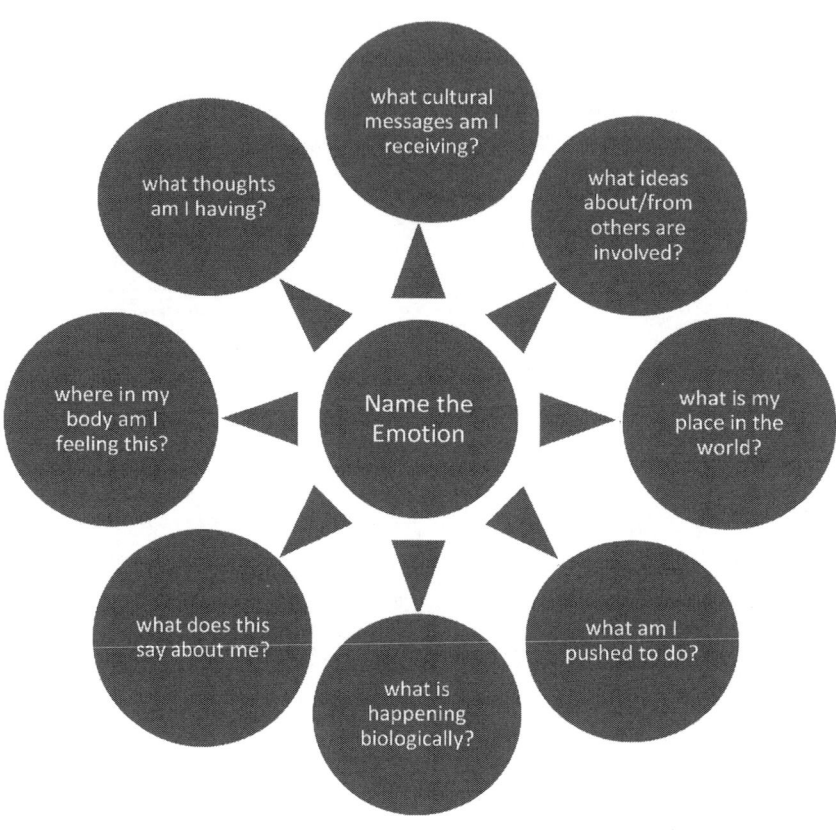

- What did you learn about yourself and your situation?

- What is important to you in how you respond?

- What would be helpful to share with your partner?

Appendix F: My partner's emotional map

Use this to imagine what your partner's emotional map may be in a particular situation. Begin with the outer circles and move toward likely emotion, thoughts, and bodily responses.

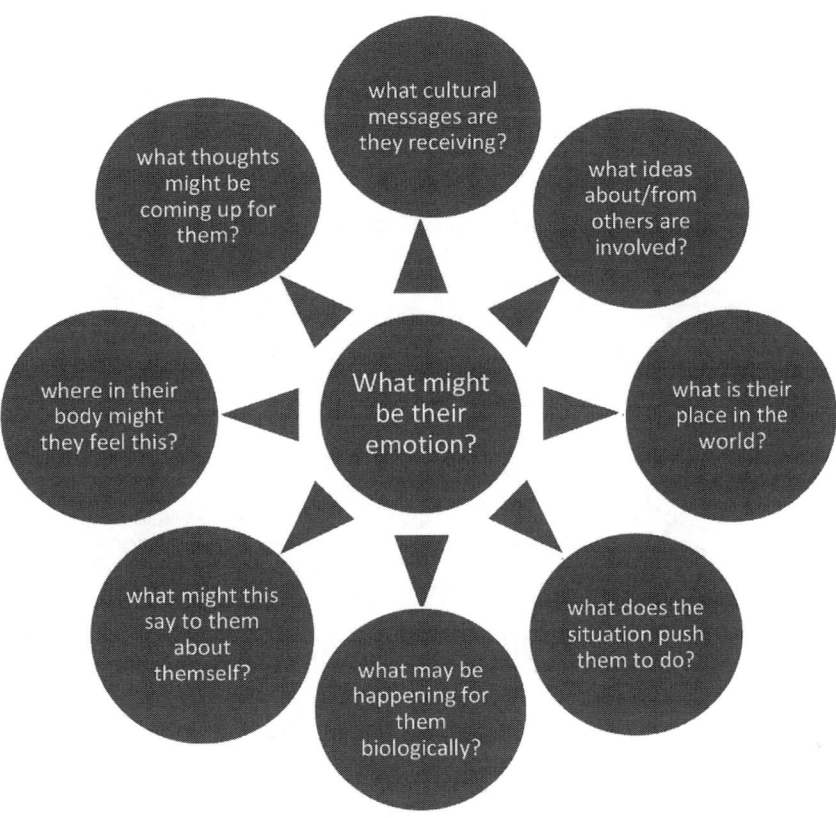

- What did you learn about your partner and their situation?

- What is likely to be important to your partner in this situation?

- What are you curious to know more about?

Appendix G: Your Relational Orientation

Below are four general ways you can orient to power and relationships. There is often a gap between the type of relationship you want and the one you have. You may also move from one orientation to another, depending on the circumstances.

- Mark an "I" next to your ideal/preferred way of orienting to your relationships
- Mark an "A" next to what is most often your actual way of relating
- Mark an "S" next to the type that emerges in conflict or stress
- Respond to the questions on the next page

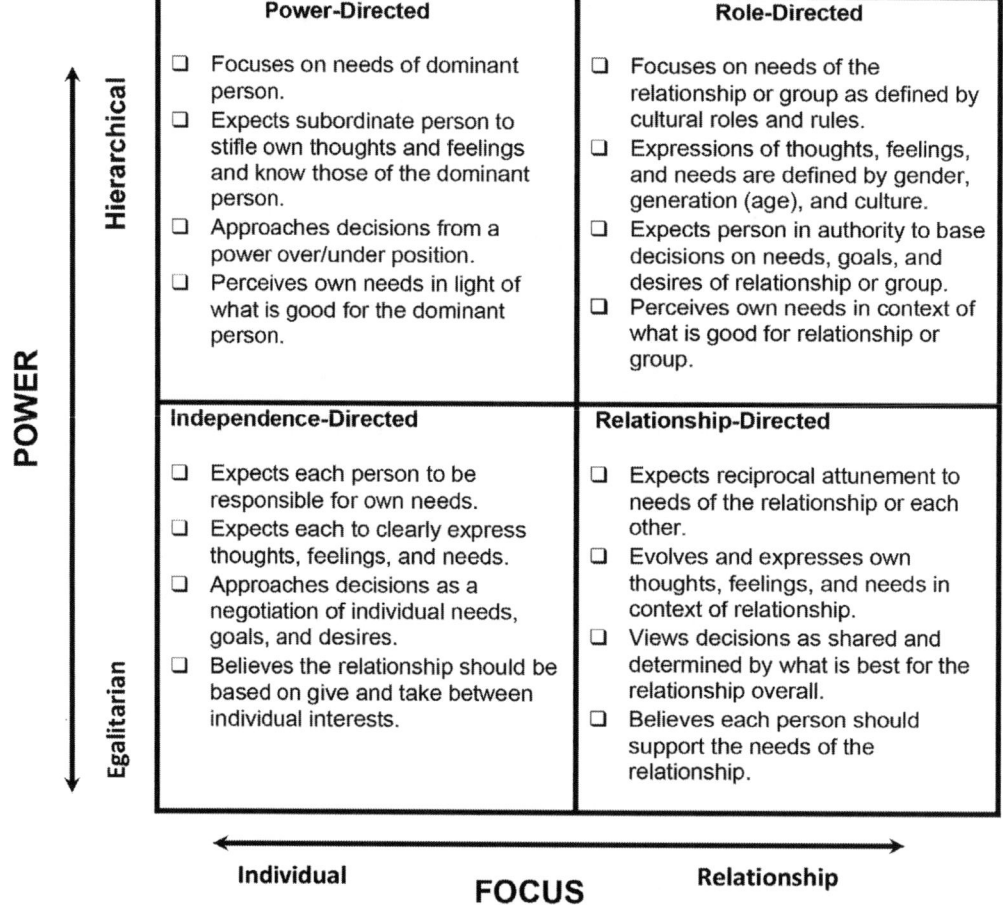

Adapted from: Silverstein, R., Bass, L. B., Tuttle, A., Knudson-Martin, C., & Huenergardt, D. (2006). What does it mean to be relational? A framework for assessment and practice. *Family Process, 45*, 391–405 (used with permission).

Reflections on your relational orientations:

1   What relational orientation did you select as your ideal? Why?

2   What interferes with your ability to orient to your relationship(s) in the way you prefer?

3   What relational orientation do you most commonly take? Is this different under conflict or stress? Does it differ from your ideal?

4   How do you and your partner(s) compare on your actual and preferred relational orientation? How do these differences and/or similarities show up in the ways you relate to each other?

5   What societal contexts and felt identities (gender, culture, etc.) affect how you orient to power and relationship?

6   Each of the relational types carries challenges in how you live together day by day. What challenges do you experience?

7   What intentional practices will help you orient to your partner from the relational type you prefer? What questions or curiosities remain?

Appendix H: Undoing Gendered Power

Patriarchy is a societal system based on male domination. It is both a mindset and the way relationships and organizations are organized. Though this system is in a process of change, the idea that men should be in charge is still active throughout society and our relationships.

Below is a list of patriarchal rules for men and boys as described by therapist and activist Rhea Almeida (2018). These rules impact everyone (male, female, queer, nonbinary). In the table below, list how you have been impacted by each rule and suggest a new rule to replace it.

The Patriarchal Male Code	*How It Has Affected Me*	*A More Equitable New Rule*
1. Don't act like a girl. Avoid and devalue "female" interests, abilities, and tasks. Project strength		
2. Keep your feelings to yourself. Don't show emotion, except anger. Vulnerability is weakness		
3. Work is your first priority. Neglect relationships and household work. Your income defines you		
4. Be self-reliant. Have answers. Make decisions on your own. Asking for help is weakness		
5. Solve problems using aggression. Be tough. Collaboration is weakness		
6. Be dominant/in control. You are either entitled to authority or accept it like a "good soldier"		
7. Women are for sex. You are entitled to sex. Sex is for your gratification or to prove your masculinity		
8. Don't be gay. Stay emotionally distant from other men. See rule 1—don't act like a girl		

What new awareness came to you as you completed this exercise?

How might you undo gendered power in your life?

Appendix I: Build Your Capacity for Mutual Vulnerability

Use this table to create a plan to enhance your capacity for mutual vulnerability. For each example of "turning toward" your partner, describe at least one new vulnerable action you will take. Do at least two each week. In the third column, describe *what you learned about yourself, your partner, and or your relationship* from doing it. Print additional copies to track your capacity over time.

Way To Turn Toward	What I Will Do & When	What I Learned
Respond to our differences or anger with curiosity about my partner's perspective		
Show self-honesty and openness about my own sensitivities		
Share what I am feeling or worried about		
Be willing to make and admit mistakes		
Ask for my partner's advice or input		
Openly express my love and caring for my partner		
Show physical affection without demands or expectations		
Show interest in my partner's life		

Notes:

Appendix J: Vulnerability and the Man Box

Mark Greene's (2018) *The Little #MeToo Book for Men* "exposes the brutal price that man box culture extracts from men and women worldwide... and invites men to step out of silence and isolation and into a better future" (back cover). The book is short, inexpensive, and easy to read. I highly recommend it.

Below is a quote from the book. Use it as a stimulus to reflect on "the man box" and mutual vulnerability:

> Go to any middle school or high school classroom in America. Ask the boys to tell you the rules for being a man. They'll all tell you the same things. Always be tough. Always be successful. Always be confident. Always have the last word. Always be the leader. But one of the first rules of manhood these boys will tell you is that "real men" don't show their emotions... to this day we coach our sons to present a façade of emotional toughness and our daughters to admire this façade in men.
>
> (p. 20)

What feelings does this statement raise for you about your experience of masculinity?

How have you been impacted by the Man Box?

What new rules do you think are needed for healthy boys, men, and relationships?

What will these new rules for men mean in your life?

Appendix K: Steps to Mutual Attunement

For each step, write an example of what you do when you successfully enact this step.

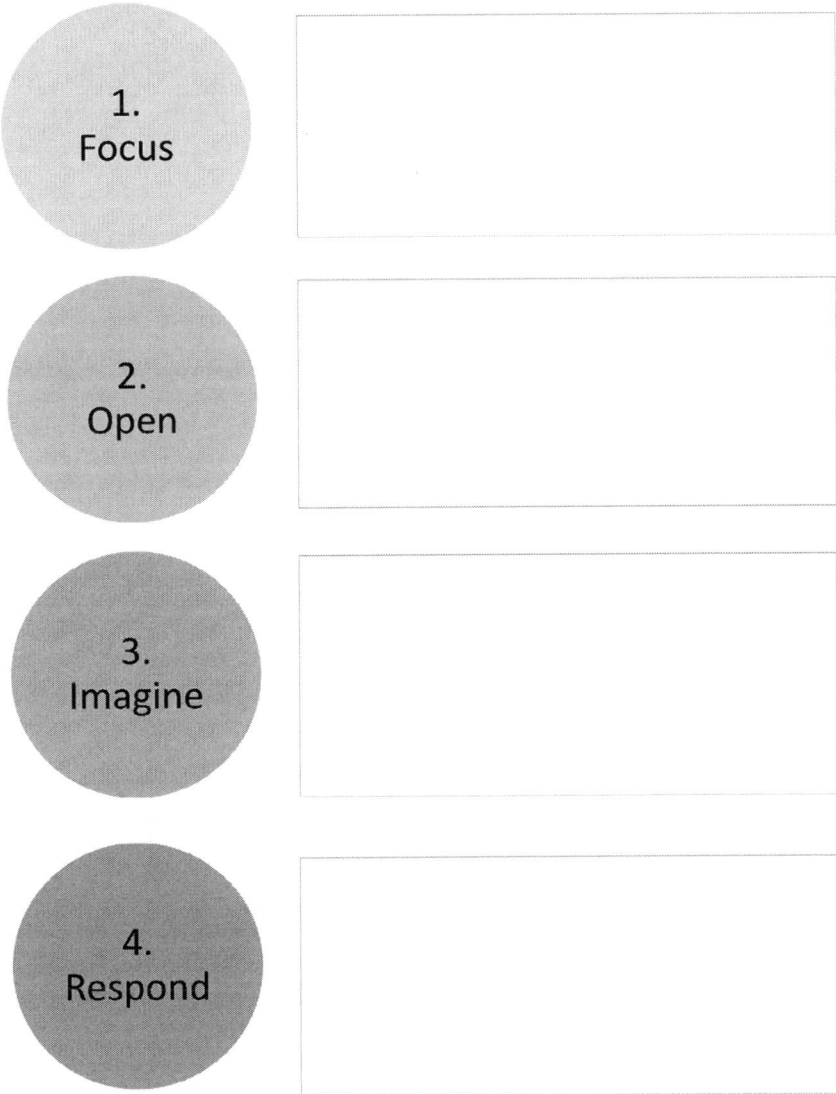

Appendix L: Openness to Influence Tracker

Use this worksheet to raise awareness about when you are open to influence from your partner (or not) and how this affects each of you. For three days, observe each of the listed areas of influence. Notice what you do and feel. Note the effect on you and your partner.

Area Of Influence	What You Did	What You Felt	Effect On You And Your Partner
Your partner was able to engage you in addressing a topic or issue of interest or concern to them	Day 1		
	Day 2		
	Day 3		
You noticed what you partner was feeling or needed and supportively responded	Day 1		
	Day 2		
	Day 3		
You changed your schedule or what you did to fit your partners' needs, interests, or suggestions	Day 1		
	Day 2		
	Day 3		

What patterns did you notice about your openness to influence?

What is the effect of your openness to influence (or lack of it) on your partner and relationship?

How would your partner's observations of their openness to influence from you be similar or different?

What new awareness or commitment arises for you as a result of these observations?

Appendix M: Our Plan to Share Relational Responsibility

Sharing relational responsibility is more than a checklist. It begins with a relational mindset and commitment to "we," and also involves intentional planning to move beyond old rules that place responsibility for relationships and care work on women. **This plan needs to be a cooperative effort, developed together.**

1. Write a statement that describes your commitment to sharing responsibility for the relationship and care work.

2. Use the chart below to (a) identify specific care and relationship maintenance tasks that need to be done, including those that usually remain behind the scenes; (b) determine how you will divide this work, who will take the lead? How will you cooperate? And (c) picture what you will see when this relational work is shared.

What Needs To Be Done: List The Tasks	How To Divide The Work: Who Takes The Lead? When?	What You Will See When Responsibility Is Shared
Child/elder care: List who needs care Direct caregiving (*feeding, bathing, dressing/changing, etc.*) Helping/coaching (*reading to, homework, skill development, reminding of schedules and chores, etc.*) Insuring safety and well-being (*monitoring activities, calming emotions, providing comfort and support, anticipating and preventing risks, etc.*) Driving/escorting (*taking to school/bus, activities, appointments, etc.*) Arranging services (*babysitters, in-home care, haircuts, scheduling, etc.*) Buying clothes and supplies Other child/elder tasks (list)		
What Needs To Be Done: List The Tasks	*How To Divide The Work: Who Takes The Lead? When?*	*What You Will See When Responsibility Is Shared*
Connections with people you care about: List names of family members, friends Checking in (*thinking about, texting, phone calls, greeting cards, etc.*) Making arrangements (*planning get-togethers/ activities, etc.*) Remembering (*tracking and responding to birthdays, important life events/activities, etc.*) Other connections tasks (*list*)		

What Needs To Be Done: *List The Tasks*	*How To Divide The Work: Who Takes The Lead? When?*	*What You Will See When Responsibility Is Shared*

Pets: list names
  Feeding (*buying pet's food, feeding, etc.*)
  Exercise and daily health (*walking or providing access to healthy environment, bathing, brushing, etc.*)
  Cleaning up (*cleaning messes, cages, tanks, etc.*)
  Veterinary care (*finding and arranging needed care*)
  Other pet tasks (*list*)		

Food
  Planning (what to cook, who likes what, allergies, what staples and ingredients to buy)
  Shopping (*buying groceries, staples, take-out, etc.*)
  Cooking (*food preparation*)
  Clean Up (*clearing table and kitchen, washing dishes, filling/emptying dishwasher*)
  Other food tasks (*list*)		

What Needs To Be Done: *List The Tasks*	*How To Divide The Work: Who Takes The Lead? When?*	*What You Will See When Responsibility Is Shared*

Household
  Daily tidying (*making beds, picking up, sweeping, reminding others of what needs to be done, etc.*)
  Cleaning (*Bathrooms, vacuuming, dusting, emptying trash, etc.*)
  Laundry (*gathering, washing, putting away, dry cleaning, etc.*)
  Supplies (*noticing what paper products, cleaning supplies, linens, etc., are needed, purchasing them, etc.*)
  Yardwork (*gardening, mowing lawn, weeds, trimming, etc.*)
  Garbage (*putting out/taking in, recycling, etc.*)
  Bills (*budgeting, tracking expenses, managing accounts, paying bills, taxes, etc.*)
  Maintenance (*making or arranging for repairs, cleaners, decorating, etc.*)
  Monitoring (*noticing state of the home, what needs to be done, coordinating tasks, etc.*)
  Transportation (*arranging, attending to auto maintenance, coordinating travel schedules*)
  Other household tasks (*list*)		

What Needs To Be Done: List The Tasks	How To Divide The Work: Who Takes The Lead? When?	What You Will See When Responsibility Is Shared
Health and well-being 　Planning (*arranging health care appointments, dealing with insurance, etc.*) 　Tending (*noticing and tracking signs of illness or emotional distress, responding to needs for attention and care*) 　Supplies (*tracking and purchasing grooming and health care supplies*) 　Emergencies (*receives notifications of child or other's illness, rearranges schedule to provide care*) 　Protective activities (*supporting time for exercise, meditation, sleep, and other health-enhancing activities*) 　Other health tasks (*list*)		
What Needs To Be Done: List The Tasks	*How To Divide The Work: Who Takes The Lead? When?*	*What You Will See When Responsibility Is Shared*
Our relationship 　Time (*how we coordinate, how we schedule, whose time matters, etc.*) 　Planning (*suggesting and arranging activities together, looking ahead to family/relationship interests, etc.*) 　Emotional climate (*monitors and attends to the mood of the relationship, calms yourself so you can attend to other, etc.*) 　Tending (*Noticing and responding to partner's emotional needs and personal concerns/activities, monitoring how you impact them, etc.*) 　Repairing (*noticing when something is wrong and initiating efforts to address them, accountability for impact on partner, etc.*) 　Sharing (*letting partner know what is important to me, asking about and listening to other, etc.*) 　We focus. (*thinking about the relationship overall, how we prioritize and cooperate, our relational goals, considering what our "we" needs*) 　Other relationship tasks (*list*)		

3.　How will you check in with each other to determine how shared responsibility for the relationship is going and what changes you may need to make? Write your agreement below.

Appendix N: How to Create Your Picture of "We"

Working together to create a picture of "we" enables you to express values and emotional sentiments that you might not otherwise articulate. It gives a tangible expression of what matters to you as a couple that you can see and draw upon. Below are two examples. You do NOT need to be an artist to do these.

1   Use pictures and/or words to create an image that symbolically represents your "we."

   a   Use any materials you like (i.e., pictures from magazines, photos, colored pens, paints, drawings, computer-generated graphics, etc.) to symbolize what matters to you in your relationship, the principles you live by.
   b   As you select the images, discuss what they mean to each of you. Work together to identify and represent concepts that you agree upon.
   c   On a piece of paper, canvas, or other frameable material, arrange your images to create a collage or representation of who you are as a couple. Share with each other what this commitment means to you and represents for your future.
   d   Place your completed "Our Picture of We" where you can readily see it.

2   Use shadow boxes to make an altar that express what is meaningful to you as a couple. *Altares*, as they are called in Spanish, are especially significant in Latino, Indigenous, Catholic, and Afro-Caribbean cultures as a way to publicly honor important relationships.

   a   Make or purchase a wooden frame or shadow box within which you will glue items that represent your picture of "we."
   b   Gather items that are meaningful to you when you think about the values and commitments at the core of your relationship (use figurines, pictures from magazines, small objects, documents, etc.)
   c   As you decide on which items to use and where to place them in the shadowbox, discuss what they mean to you and what say about who you are as a couple and your commitment to "we."
   d   Place your shadow box in a visible place as a public commitment to each other. As you do, reiterate the values that your picture of "we" represents.

Source: Bermúdez, J. M. & Bermúdez, S. (2002). Altar-making with Latino families: A narrative therapy perspective. Journal of Family Psychotherapy, 13(3/4). Reprinted in T. D. Carlson and M. J. Erickson (Eds), Spirituality and Family Therapy. Haworth Press.

Appendix O: Guidelines for SERT Group Reflections

The Socio-Emotional Relationship Workbook for Couples helps you develop a new story about intimate relationships. Groups are an ideal way to develop and solidify this new narrative.

The guidelines below emphasize how group members can co-create new relational meanings as they tell their own stories and witness and reflect on those of others, while avoiding debate and judgment. They may be applied in a variety of group formats.

(A) When you are the speaker, share your story/perspective as openly as possible. Accept the genuine interest and curiosity of your witnesses.

(B) When you are a witness do not:

   - make judgments or evaluations (good or bad)
   - tell moral stories
   - give advice

(C) When you are a witness, do:

   - Share images in teller's stories that evoked a response in you
   - Share what resonated with you personally
   - Share what touched you

   (This is not how people usually respond to one another)

(D) Four kinds of reflections are especially helpful.

   1 What the speaker said that gave you a sense of what the person values or holds dear, especially those connected to relationships and/or how they want to be seen
   2 Images that come to your mind as the speaker talks and what they *might* reflect on this person's unique dreams and aspirations—always offer these tentatively
   3 What struck a chord with your own personal history and relational struggles
   4 What moved you as a result of witnessing these stories:

      - a new perspective on your own life
      - something you hadn't thought of for awhile
      - new meanings that come to you
      - new steps you might be prompted to take

(E) The speaker is asked to reflect on what they are drawn to from the feedback. This back and forth helps create new shared meaning.

Guidelines adapted from reflecting principles suggested by Michael White (2007) in *Maps of Narrative Practice*.

Appendix P: BEST Conversations Format for Difficult Topics

Phase I **B**ecome **P**resent	(A) Agree on an amount of time for getting in touch with yourself and becoming present. Take at least five minutes.
	(B) Silently review your emotion maps (Appendix E) as they relate to the topic you are about to discuss.
	(C) Close your eyes, make yourself comfortable, and take slow, deep breathes in…and out…
	(D) As you continue to gently breathe in and out, picture yourself within expanding circles of relationships. Be aware of your partner… your places of belonging… how you know yourself in the world.
	(E) As you breathe in and out, let yourself be present to the topic for discussion. Be aware of tensions you feel around this subject… where you feel them in your body… what shoulds/oughts or right/wrongs are present… what these say about you and what matters to you.
	(F) As you continue to gently breathe in and out, let these tensions relax. Let them "be." Be aware of your partner and your interest in their perspectives… in what matters to them.
	(G) As you continue to slowly breathe in and out, orient yourself to learning with curiosity and openness to new awareness and possibilities.

Phase II
Expand **M**utual
Awareness

Format for Structured Conversation

- Each of you responds to the first question for two minutes. When you are talking, take time to let your thinking evolve but do not speak longer than two minutes.
- When one of you is speaking, the other(s) does not interrupt or comment. When you are listening, focus on your partner. Resist the urge to [even silently] question, add, disagree, etc.
- Move on to the next question, repeating the format.
- When the impulse to directly answer or debate each other arises, gently and respectfully remind yourselves to return to the structured process.

Awareness Questions

1 Share a story that shows why [this topic] is important to you. The story (or stories) may be from any time and place in your life. Explain what about this story is meaningful to you.

2 What messages related to your felt identities (gender, race/ethnicity, class, sexuality, abilities, etc.) come up around [this topic]? What do they say you should think, feel, or do? Where do these messages come from?

3 When [this topic] comes up between you, what is your fear or worry? How do you experience this fear? What does it say about you and/or the situation? Use your emotion map as a guide.

4 When [this topic] comes up between you, what is your hope or dream? What does this dream mean to you? Use your emotion map as a guide.

5 What are you uncertain or confused about regarding [this topic]? What are you flexible about? Explain.

6   As you listen to your own and your partner's responses to these questions, what new awareness, ideas, or questions come up for you? What would you like to know more about? (partner does not answer)

7   What will it mean to you when [this topic] brings less trouble or division between you? What will it say about your relationship? About you? About you partner? Explain.

Repeat the sequence again following the same format. This enables you to build upon and expand beyond your initial responses. Use again as needed.

Phase III
Seek New
Options

A.   Brainstorm. Let ideas flow with minimum discussion. Use Appendix P to record your thoughts and ideas. It has three "pots" for your thoughts and ideas.

Pot 1: list take-aways from your previous conversation
Pot 2: list possible agreements/solutions—no matter how silly they may seem
Pot 3: list small changes that could matter

Make additions to any of these lists as you think of them

B.   Discuss and organize your brainstormed lists.
What jumps out at you?
Where is there overlap?
What is new that you didn't see before?
Explore how specific possibilities might work.
Don't rush to agreement—leave room to discuss without commitment

C.   Make a temporary agreement.

Agree to cooperate on something. It could be as simple as agreeing to disagree, a small first step that each of you are willing to take, or a new shared vision of what cooperation around this issue looks like.

Phase IV
Trust You Will
Work Through
Challenges

A.   Expect new challenges will arise
B.   Commit to work through them together
C.   Commit to relationality, equity, and mutual support through the Circle of Care
D.   Evolve as you and your circumstances change

Appendix Q: BEST Brainstorming Record

To generate new options, brainstorm in each of the following "pots." Keep discussion to a minimum until brainstorming is complete. Record each of your ideas and thoughts regardless of how "silly." Use another page if necessary.

Pot 1—Take-Aways From Your Previous Conversation	Pot 2—Possible Agreements/ Solutions	Pot 3—Small Changes That Could Matter

References

Almeida, R. V. (2018). *Liberation based healing practices*. The Institute for Family Services.

Bava, S. & Greene, M. (2023). *The relational workplace: How relational intelligence grows diverse, equitable, and inclusive cultures of connection*. ThinkPlay Partners.

Bermúdez, J. M. & Bermúdez, S. (2002). Altar-making with Latino families: A narrative therapy perspective. *Journal of Family Psychotherapy*, 13(3/4). Reprinted in T. D. Carlson and M. J. Erickson (Eds), *Spirituality and Family Therapy*. Haworth Press.

Coontz, S. (2005). *Marriage, a history: From obedience to intimacy or how love conquered marriage*. Viking.

Cowdery, R., S., Scarborough, N., Lewis, M. E., & Seshadri, G. (2009). Pulling together How African American couples manage social inequalities. In C. Knudson-Martin & A. R. Mahoney (Eds), *Couples, gender, and power: Creating change in intimate relationships* (pp. 215–233). Springer Publishing Co.

Damasio, A. R. (1994). *Descartes' error: Emotion, reason, and the human brain*. Quill.

Dolan-Del Vecchio, K. (2008). *Making love, playing power: Men, women and the rewards of intimate justice*. Soft Skull Press.

Fishbane, Mona (2013). *Loving with the brain in mind: Neurobiology & couple therapy*. Norton.

Gottman, J. M. (2011). *The science of trust: Emotional attunement for couples*. Norton.

Greene, M. (2018). *The Little #MeToo Book for Men*. ThinkPlay Partners.

Herman, J. L. (2023). *Truth and repair: How trauma survivors envision justice*. Basic Books.

Jonathan, N. (2009). Carrying equal weight: Relational responsibility and attunement among same-sex couple. In C. Knudson-Martin & . A. R. Mahoney (Eds), *Couples, gender, and power: Creating change in intimate relationships* (pp. 79–103). Springer Publishing Co.

Knudson-Martin, C. (2024). *A step-by-step guide to socio-emotional relationship therapy: A socially responsible approach to clinical practice*. Routledge.

Knudson-Martin, C., Kim, L., Gibbs, E., & Harmon, R. (2021). Sociocultural attunement to vulnerability in couple therapy: Fulcrum for changing power processes. *Family Process*, 60, 1152–1169.

Knudson-Martin, C. & Mahoney, A. R. (Eds) (2009). *Couples, gender, and power: Creating change in intimate relationships*. Springer Publishing Co.

McDowell, T., Knudson-Martin, C., & Bermudez, J. M. (2023). *Socioculturally attuned family therapy: Guidelines for equitable theory and practice* (2nd ed.). Routledge.

Pandit, M., Kang, Y. J., ChenFeng, J., Knudson-Martin, C., & Huenergardt D. (2014). Practicing socio-cultural attunement: A study of couple therapists. *Journal of Contemporary Family Therapy*, 36, 518–528.

Rodsky, E. (2019). *Fair play: Share the mental lead, rebalance your relationship and transform your life*. Quercus.

Schore, A. (2021). The interpersonal neurobiology of intersubjectivity. *Frontiers in Psychology*, 12, 648616. doi:10.3389/fpsyg.2021.648616.

Siegel, D. J. (2020). *The developing mind: How relationships and the brain interact to shape who we are* (3rd ed.). Guilford Press.

Silverstein, R., Bass, L. B., Tuttle, A., Knudson-Martin, C., Huenergardt, D. (2006). What does it mean to be relational? A framework for assessment and practice. *Family Process*, 45, 391–405.

Skerrett, K. (2022). *Growing married: Creating stories for a lifetime of love*. LifeCycle Press.

Tichenor, V. J. (2005). *Earning more and getting less: Why successful wives can't buy equality*. Rutgers University Press.

U.S. Surgeon General's advisory on the healing effects of social connection and community (2023). Our epidemic of loneliness and isolation. www.hhs.gov/sites/default/files/surgeon-general-social-connection-advisory.pdf.

Waldinger, R. & Schulz, M. (2023). *The good life: Lessons from the world's longest scientific study of happiness*. Simon & Schuster.

Way, N., Ali, A., Gilligan, C., & Noguera, P. (Eds). (2018). *The crisis of connection: Roots, consequences, and solutions*. NYU Press.

White, M. (2007). *Maps of narrative practice*. Norton.

9781032759890